Ron's Story

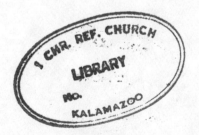

Ron's Story
A Legacy of Love

By Marie Butler

GOOD NEWS PUBLISHERS
Westchester, Illinois 60153

*To my family
for their love and understanding during
the bad times; for their laughter and
wonderful sense of humor that made the
good times. They made me a*
LIBERATED WOMAN
*Others have more beauty, talent—
And lead a more interesting life.
But if I were any other woman,
I wouldn't be my husband's wife.
I wouldn't want to be someone else;
Nor do I envy another.
For if I weren't who I am,
I wouldn't be my children's mother.*

RON'S STORY
A Legacy of Love

Copyright © 1978 by Marie Butler
*All rights reserved.
Printed in the United States of America.*

Library of Congress Catalog Card Number 78-52686
ISBN 0-89107-155-5

*We gratefully acknowledge the following for
permission to reprint copyrighted material:*
Grit *magazine* © *1975 for "Liberated Woman."*

Contents

Prologue / 7

Part I Starting Over

Chapter 1 The "Perfect Mother" Complex / 17

Chapter 2 Cowboy Hats and Clown Smiles / 23

Chapter 3 Back Seat Beauticians / 29

Chapter 4 It Can't Happen to Us / 37

Part II Ron's Story

Chapter 5 The Beginning of the End / 51

Chapter 6 A Time to Laugh, a Time to Cry / 59

Chapter 7 A Sign of Hope / 71

Chapter 8 Buying Time / 83

Chapter 9 Nuggets of Gold / 95

Chapter 10 For Everything There Is a Season / 109

Chapter 11 Grief / 127

Epilogue / 139

Prologue

In 1947 I stood on the bank of a rampaging river near my parents' farm. "God," I shouted, "I'm so sick of this rotten world, but I don't have the courage to leave it. I'm a failure. Sometimes—most of the time—I hate myself and everyone else."

One leap into the flooded river would end 22 years of conflicts from an ugly-duckling childhood and an acne-faced adolescence, to an adult who couldn't face up to the failure of her marriage.

As long as God said "yes" to all my prayers and life ran smoothly, I could manage. But when the testing got rough, I cried, "God . . . help me! I'm so scared. Give me one reason why I shouldn't jump. Give me some reason for living."

The wind snuffed out my pleading voice as the child beneath my heart moved, jerking my mind back from thoughts of death. My collie dog whined softly as I fell to the ground beside him and cried myself out on his soft neck. He touched my arm with his paw as though he understood.

Pal had been given to us when his master went off to war; now he didn't want him back. "Poor old fellow," I cried in his ear. "We're two of a kind. We don't really belong anywhere."

Our family moved often during my childhood, making me forever the outsider and giving me a very unstable feeling with my peers and teachers. Being the only girl and the youngest didn't help. Dad and Mom had each other. My two brothers, only a year apart, had each other. It seemed as though I fit in only when they had a difference of opinion. Whether imagined or real, I grew up feeling rejected. Growing up with the nickname "Pest" and never really belonging to any religion or community made me feel as though I walked alone around an invisible circle I couldn't penetrate.

My mother was the only person I could talk to, but the demands on her time and energy didn't leave her much time, so I learned to talk to Jesus.

Early in life I had a fear of God. It was not a healthy fear—more like that of a strict disciplinarian who would punish me severely at the slightest provocation. But as I grew older and learned about Jesus, I came to know Him as a friend, one I could talk to—sometimes the only friend I had.

With covers over my head, so Dad or my brothers wouldn't make fun of me, I would sob out my hurts to Him. His love would comfort me, giving me hope. But Satan was usually close by, working through people or circumstances, to push me nearer the brink of self-destruction.

Another gentle kick from my baby broke the depression. A calmness came over me as if Jesus were standing beside me. Pal and I started across the fields toward home as the sun broke through the clouds promising a change in the gloomy weather. A rainbow arched over the pasture as playful colts celebrated the change.

Mom looked at me with concern when I went into the kitchen. "I was worried about you. I wish you wouldn't go near the river when it's like this." Mom was petrified of water, especially when it was tearing at its banks like it had been all week. There was no need to tell her where I'd been.

"Pal and I went for a walk," I said, catching a glimpse of my bloated body in the mirror. Pregnancy hadn't brought forth that inner glow of beauty that magazines were always talking about. A tall thin girl had been replaced by a tall fat woman. The skinny girl had laughed often in spite of down days. But this poor misshapen creature glaring back at me had very few things to laugh about.

No wonder my husband, Bob, said he hated the sight of pregnant women. The term male chauvinist wasn't around then, but that was a perfect description of Bob. Among the many things he had failed to tell me before our marriage was his dislike of children. His reaction to my pregnancy was: "Either have an abortion or we're through." When I refused, he agreed to let me stay until I started to show. "You can go to your parents until the kid arrives," he said. It's little wonder so many marriages fail. Most people give more thought to buying a car than picking a mate. I'm sure Bob did.

The week before I boarded a bus for home, I asked Bob to attend church with me. "Only stupid people go to church," he said. "Religion is a crutch used by weaklings like you. God, Santa Claus and the Easter bunny are all the same. You get what you want in this world by taking it—not by talking to some mystery man in the sky."

I spent most of the week alone in a hotel room while Bob gambled. It was a sickness with him. He couldn't stop—he didn't want to.

Finally, on the last morning, I walked to the bus station alone and bought a one-way ticket back to Missouri. Bob had gambled all night, sure this time he would make a "killing." He had. He'd just killed our marriage. There was no way I would bring a child up in the conditions I was leaving. I'd always dreaded the ending of relationships, but this time I didn't feel anything except that somehow I'd failed. And I wasn't quite sure what I'd failed at.

After I returned to my parents' home, fear of my unsure future took over. And Satan fed on my insecurity like an unseen vulture. I was still wrapped up in the old fear that a woman who fails at marriage will keep on failing. Fear of living was what led me to the river. I'm sure the fear of dying made me cry out to God for help. I had yet to learn that God will give help in His time and in His way. And He had a special way of casting out my terror of childbirth.

Although I read every book I could find about childbirth, I was still facing my baby's birth with panic. Mom had protected me too much. After all the years on a farm, I had never seen anything born. One day I missed our cat. I searched for hours and finally found her in the cellar. My fears fell away as I watched the miracle of birth before me. The cat and I spent all afternoon in the cellar. She had four babies, and I was awed at how she seemed to know exactly what to do. Perhaps it was a strange place to pray for my coming child. I'm sure the

Lord understood my pleading.

I went to the hospital on Christmas night. Mom stayed by my side through the night and late into the next day until darkness closed over me. A dream sent me into a valley searching wildly for my child. Instead of a baby, I found a small deer. It was making strange rasping sounds. I cried, "Oh, God, why did he die?"

Mom's voice pleaded with me as I fought my way out of the darkness. "Honey, your baby is fine. But how did you know it was a boy?"

When they placed Ronnie in my arms, I couldn't believe that tiny squirming bit of humanity was my son. His little mouth nuzzled against me and I felt important for the first time in my life. And for another first, I thanked God for the privilege of being a woman. Until then, I hadn't liked being female.

The baby was two months old when I started making plans for our future. There hadn't been a divorce in our family, and it was hoped one could be avoided. My decision came about by accident or a quick answer to prayer.

I didn't believe in divorce, but I felt my first duty was to my baby. He hadn't asked to be brought into this world. Now that he was here, I wanted him to have a good life. Fighting parents don't produce a happy home, and I was not going to turn myself into a mute servant like Bob wanted. I'd seen too much of this.

Remarks I'd heard from my own family about divorced women kept coming to mind. Criticism bothered me, but I had to take it constantly from Bob, so I was going to get it no matter what my choice. *Lord, I'm not asking for my sake but my son's. Help me make the right decision.*

Dad went to town the next morning. I hadn't planned

on going, but the baby had been sick most of the night and I needed to talk to the doctor. We didn't have a telephone, so Mom suggested I'd better go just as Dad started down the drive.

Nursing a baby was going out of style then and the doctor let me know it. He told me Ronnie's colic was because I was highly emotional. There was no way I could afford the expensive product he was pushing and told him so. I left his office feeling like a rotten mother.

Dad wasn't ready to leave, so I wandered around the square looking in windows at all the wonderful toys Ronnie would have some day and wishing I'd stayed home.

I stopped by the post office to mail a package for Mom. The clerk noticed the name and asked if I wanted the mail they were holding. Before I could tell him my parents didn't get mail there, he handed me three letters addressed to Dad. I gave Dad the letters when I got in the car.

"That's odd," he said, "Why would anyone send our mail general delivery?"

"Open them," I urged. "They're addressed to you."

Dad opened one letter. "Somebody's crazy! She talks about us being together last summer. Here, see if you can make any sense out of it."

The dates and towns made it obvious who the letters were for. "Bob's using your name. He's probably in some kind of trouble." Our marriage had gone through some stormy times; now I knew it had passed the point of no return.

Divorce wasn't taken lightly by my family or friends. Many were sure I'd change my mind. My parents knew most of the reasons. But there were some things I couldn't even tell them.

Asking for child support would have been ridiculous, since Bob couldn't hold a job. All I wanted was for him to stay out of my life.

The judge granted me full custody of the baby and said, "I hope you make a better choice if you marry again."

At that moment, marriage was not in my future. I had a son to raise. No human need goes deeper or is more comforting than the knowledge that "someone needs me."

Part I
Starting Over

Chapter 1
The "Perfect Mother" Complex

It would have been hard for me to make it after my divorce if it hadn't been for my parents. We moved to the city when Ronnie was ten months old.

It scares me sometimes when I think how much hinges on circumstances. I answered a help wanted ad the day after we moved. Several men were working on a loading dock when I arrived at the mill. "Where's the office?" I asked the man nearest me.

I felt his eyes on me as I walked to the door he pointed out. I turned. Our eyes met, and strong vibrations told me this person might eventually effect my life.

After I was hired, the office workers warned, "Don't get interested in Martin. He's a confirmed bachelor."

"That's fine with me," I answered. "I'll help him stay that way."

Martin and I became good friends. He knew I had a sour outlook on life. Still, our friendship lasted. We had known each other six months when he asked me for a date. To show him where he stood, I decided to take Ronnie. Mom was shocked. "Do you think it's wise?"

"If he doesn't like children, I might as well know now. Besides," I said, hugging my squirming son, "he probably won't come back."

Ronnie was a terror. But he and Martin hit it off as though they were old friends. Before the day ended, they had made up their minds about our future. It took longer to convince me. I thought I loved Martin. More important, I liked him. But the two don't always go together.

I had qualms about marriage. There had been one failure. Now there was a child's future to consider. When I measured all the nays against the deep love between my son and this unusual man, I said "yes" to his proposal.

Martin was a big, rugged man, and so different than any I'd known. He didn't drink, smoke, or feel that men had the right to a different set of morals than women. God had thoughtfully provided him broad shoulders. And how he needed them, for I brought all my fears and hang-ups into our marriage.

Both of us were lonely souls who had resigned ourselves to never finding that special person. We had a good marriage, partly because of luck, and because we worked at it—especially Martin. He was the most understanding person I had ever known.

There were a thousand reasons why we wouldn't make it past the first year. And there was only one reason we would—we loved each other. We knew there had been bets that it wouldn't last. The house we bought was old and in need of repair. Some remarked, "The house will probably last longer than the marriage." It made me angry, but Martin didn't let it bother him.

Some of our trouble wouldn't have happened if Martin hadn't adopted Ronnie. The law wouldn't allow adoption until we had been married nine months. We saved enough for court fees and filed. The court checked with every friend and neighbor. We were not a couple with a child then; Martin was a step-father. And once it was known, I was the target of the critical tongue of my neighbor, Mary.

"After all," she pointed out, "you've failed at one marriage, there isn't much chance for a second." From then on, she criticized everything I did. If I scolded Ronnie, her eyebrows went up in an expression I learned to hate. "And Martin," she reminded me, "is only a step-father; no wonder the child is so mean."

"Can't you get it through your thick head," I screamed at her one day, "Martin will be his legal father. How many men would spend two months' pay to adopt a child they already have? That kid of yours isn't perfect, you know!"

Mary slammed out of the house. And I'm sure she was the one who started the gossip that there was no big deal to the adoption, because I hadn't been married before. Long before that lie got back to me, Bob signed the papers. When he learned the court would hold Martin responsible for the child's welfare, Bob couldn't get the papers back fast enough.

We would have been extremely happy, if I could have turned off outside interference. People just couldn't forget. It seemed to annoy some that we were happy as a family. If Martin corrected Ronnie, he was a mean step-father. If he didn't, Ronnie was a spoiled brat.

Some wanted to be sure our son knew he was adopted. One evening we were visiting relatives when Ronnie flung himself into Martin's arms. "Oh, Daddy," he sobbed, "the kids said you were mean and ran off and left me."

"Son, I wouldn't leave you," Martin said, hugging the bewildered child.

"It's time for us to go," I said, trying to hold my temper.

On the way home, I questioned Ronnie about what the girls had told him. "They said my daddy was mean and ran away because he didn't like me." He reached over and clutched Martin's arm. "You do like me, don't you, Daddy?"

Martin pulled the car off the road. Tears were blinding him as he took Ronnie from me. "I love you, Son. Don't ever let anyone tell you different." Turning to me, he whispered, "Those little stinkers need a spanking."

There had been several adoptions in Martin's family. They accepted Ronnie as one of the clan. But it was not going to be that way with my relatives. "They were only repeating what their parents told them," I said. "From now on we'll stay away."

We loved remodeling our old house and working in the yard. Ronnie and I rescued wild flowers from areas marked for new housing projects. His tiny fingers would plant violets in every spare corner, then he would explain to Pal that he'd better not dig there.

Pal was not a city dog. The over-sized ancient collie belonged on a farm. But he was no longer useful to anyone except Ronnie. There had always been a strong bond between them. Pal had never had a small boy to play with and was making up for lost time. A walk in the fields beyond our house could last for hours, and there was always a gift of wild flowers, a rock or a leaf for me.

There were so many times when we didn't know whether to laugh, cry, or spank. Like the day Martin decided to paint the house and Ronnie wanted to help. Patient Daddy helped the little hand grip the paint brush and together they painted a lower section. After the novelty wore off, Ronnie came in the house for a drink.

A neighbor called Martin over to help him on his car. I went out to tell them dinner was ready as Martin came in the gate. "Where's Ronnie?" I asked.

"Isn't he inside? He was when I left."

"I'm painting," was all we needed to send us running around the house. He had painted the ladder, windows, the dog, and himself. The rest of my day was devoted to cleaning up the boy and dog. Martin cleaned paint off of the windows, but the ladder would always be a reminder to never leave an open paint bucket near little boys.

Ronnie was three when our baby, Kathy, joined us. As I held my little girl for the first time, I asked God for the wisdom and whatever else it took to raise children in our circumstances and not have the word adoption haunt us. Her birth also reminded me of the foreboding dream I'd had about Ronnie at his birth. I tried to shove it to the back of my mind, but never completely succeeded.

Kathy was a good baby. But somewhere along the way I picked up a "perfect mother" complex. It's so easy for a person to get bogged down in the pressure of daily living. How are we going to stretch this week's pay to cover the emergency doctor bill or car repairs? How come my yard is full of kids and dogs when I have two children and one dog? Someone is hurt, dogs are fighting, the phone is ringing and so on until sometimes the load gets too heavy.

Chapter 2
Cowboy Hats and Clown Smiles

There will always be days that fade the bloom from a mother's disposition—you know the kind I mean: the alarm didn't go off and Martin was late for work; Kathy dumped a bowl of cereal in her lap; after the floor was clean and waxed, Ronnie let the dog in out of the rain.

Days like that had a tendency to jolt my perspective, making me wonder where I'd gone wrong. Parenthood was something I had looked upon as instinct which would magically appear when needed. It wasn't. It hadn't. And it didn't. I ranted and raved at the wrong times, laughed in the wrong places, and felt like a complete failure as a mother.

Child psychology was a big thing in the early fifties—at least it seemed that way to me. We read Doctor Spock and every child-care expert we heard about.

After putting the baby down for a nap, I poured a cup of coffee and decided to check with Doctor Spock to see where . . . "Hey lady," a voice called, "there's a fire in your basement!"

A meter reader was grinning up at me as I ran out the door. "In there by the furnace."

There sat Ronnie roasting marshmallows. "Pal wanted some," he yelled, as I put out the fire.

Forgetting all the educated advice, and my good intentions, I spanked him. As I sent the sticky boy upstairs, the dog slinked out the door.

By the time Ronnie was clean, he had cleared the air with hugs, kisses and plain old flattery. No mother can resist bribes when they come in the form of, "You're the bestest mommy in the whole world."

"Don't you leave the porch," I warned, as I started dinner. It wasn't long before Martin came home. Pal barked loud enough to jar my aching head, and Ronnie made a flying leap into his daddy's arms.

"Hey, when I get a welcome like that, I can bet a guy's in trouble," Martin said, hugging him.

Ronnie looked very serious. "I don't think Mommy feels good. She's had a bad day."

Trying to hide a grin, Martin came in shaking his head. "Has he been his usual self today?"

"Here," I said, handing him a spoon. "You stir while I have a nervous breakdown."

"That bad?"

I nodded, trying to hold back the tears, "I'm such a failure. How can I expect him to mind when I scream at him like a shrew?"

"Hey, you're talking about the woman I love. Stop running her down. Besides, that's not much of a welcome for a husband," he said, pulling my head down on his shoulder.

"I can't help it. How can I learn to handle my own

problems when I can't control a child?"

"He's just going through a phase, Honey. It'll pass."

It seemed as though Ronnie always found another phase to go through before I could cope with the one he'd just left. To call him an average child would be stretching the imagination beyond infinity. He was a lovable bundle of energy, a Dennis the Menace come to life. His agile little mind thought up all sorts of interesting things to do or talk about. In the middle of baking cookies, he would turn his freckled elfin face up and gaze intently at me. "Mom, what if I wasn't your kid?" "What if God forgot to turn on the sun in the morning?" His questions continued so much we called him little "What If." Sometimes the what ifs were serious because he wanted to learn. But often they were meant to be funny or delay bed time. One night he had been told "good-night" several times, when I discovered he was in the kitchen.

"Young man," I scolded, "you get into bed—now!"

"I'm hungry," he insisted, "and I forgot to look in Daddy's lunch box to see what he left me."

This was a ritual that started when Martin and I got married. There was something special about anything left in Daddy's lunch box. Although the same kind of fruit or cookies were in the cabinet, it always tasted better when found as a treasure at the end of the day. I always packed something extra each morning. The few times Martin was hungry and ate everything, he stopped by the store to replace it.

As Ronnie ate the apple he had found, I asked him why he couldn't sleep. "There's too many things to do," he said, "and Bear keeps me awake."

"Now you listen to me, Bear," I scolded, shaking my finger at the stuffed toy clutched in Ronnie's arms. "You get in bed and tell Ronnie stories."

There was a big pretense of giving Bear a bit of apple. "What if there's a Martian hiding under my bed? . . . Or a mean ghost? . . . Or a . . ." He stopped, and with a mischievous grin looked up at my scowling face. "I think I'm sleepy now," he said, hurrying to his room.

Kathy, a tiny golden blonde, with the dispoisiton of an angel, usually followed her brother into all his trouble and adventures. A large box could be a wagon taking them across the prairie, a pirate ship or a space ship flying to the moon. Pal and Fluffy, the family cat, were always part of the crew.

No matter how good my intentions, I didn't always have the children cleaned up when Martin came home. It didn't bother him, even though Mary tactfully pointed out that my children sometimes looked like urchins.

When I apologized one night, Martin pulled me down beside him on the grass.

"Look at them," he scolded. "It would be mean to stop their play now."

"I know, but sometimes I wish I could be more like other mothers."

"I hope you don't mean Mary."

"She always has everything on schedule, everything so neat. I guess she is just more efficient than I am."

"Mary would be the first to agree. In fact, she probably told you that. How did things go today?"

"Fair," I sighed. "But you know me, try . . . try . . . try . . . No matter what I do it doesn't seem good enough."

"Stop that! Why are you always putting yourself down?"

Blinking back tears that came too easily, I added, "I've been conditioned to it. I'm constantly overwhelmed by small problems that don't bother other people. When are you going to realize you married a loser?"

Martin put his arm around my shoulders. "Honey, an old proverb says: 'There is only one beautiful child in the world and every mother has it.' Can you look at our two little imps and say you're a loser? Don't you know that you have more love from the three of us than some women will ever know?"

Through my tears, I watched our children building a fort. Their bare feet looked as though they hadn't seen shoes or water for a week. Kathy's face had streaks of dirt where tears had trickled when she fell from her play horse. Her long hair had slipped from its ponytail. An old cowboy hat was perched on Ronnie's unruly hair. Both had huge Kool-Aid clown smiles around their lips. They were happy. Why couldn't I bury the past and tune out critics?

The past haunted me, the future scared me and I was unable to deal with the present. I needed help, but the few people I had turned to made me feel guilty.

"A good Christian need only pray," I was told. "If you would . . ." It seemed everyone knew what I should or shouldn't do except me.

whether to shout, "Rejoice, that dead body is our
people. When are you going to realize you married a
hero?"

Mocha put his arm around my shoulder. "I love all
our two embassy. There is not one beautiful child in the
world and every mother has it. Can you look at our two
little ones and say you don't love them? Don't you know that
you have more love than the three of us men their
women will ever know."

Through his tears, I watched our children building a
fort. Their once taut looks as though they hadn't seen
shoes or water for a week. Kathy, who had stood up to
her whatevers, had melted when she fell from her play
horse. Her long hair had flopped from its ponytail. An
old cowboy hat was perched on Kevin's sullenly bare
flesh, and little Kosa-Anh thrown grudges around the tips.
They were happy. Who could rob! Bury the past and try
our critics?

The past taunted me, the future stared ahead, and I was
unable to deal with the present. I needed help, but the
few people I had turned to made me feel guilty.

"A good Christian need only pray," I was told. "If
you would ..." It seemed everyone knew what I
should or shouldn't do except me.

Chapter 3
Back Seat Beauticians

Family traditions are what memories are made of. We started early to develop our own. I could remember the confusion in my own childhood concerning Jesus' birthday and Santa Claus—the Resurrection and Easter bunnies. It was hard for me to understand why Santa left more toys at my friend's house than mine. Especially when most of my friends were just as ornery as I was.

Martin and I thought the emphasis on Santa and the Easter bunny was overdone. I was trying to think of a way to explain it when Ronnie simplified things on Kathy's first Christmas.

"Are we going to tell her that story about Santa?" he asked, as we decorated the tree.

"Do you think we should?" I said, prying tinsel from Kathy's fingers.

He looked at the baby, then at the fireplace. "I guess it'll be all right while she's little. But I know that fat old man can't come down our chimney."

That was the Christmas Ronnie became upset because there wasn't a birthday cake for dinner. I thought he had Christmas and his birthday confused and assured him he would have a cake the next day. "But Jesus should have a birthday cake," he cried.

It's hard to explain to a four year old why mother doesn't have time to do something. But he was delighted the next day to have turkey left over from Jesus' birthday. "Isn't this nice to have a party for Jesus one day and have all this left for my party?" he asked. I vowed that from now on there would be a cake for both birthdays.

We wanted our children to know the true reason behind each holiday and be on a one-to-one basis with the Lord. Bedtime prayers sometimes grew into a lengthy conversation with Him, forming a habit we would be grateful for later. I wanted them to know Jesus as a loving companion, not as the strict disciplinarian figure I had feared as a child. As with most child-rearing theories, we would not know the results of our teaching until the children were older.

One of my best lessons on parenthood came about because I stopped by a children's home to leave quilts from our church. A beautiful cake was on the hall table. It was made in the form of an old fashioned girl. The actual cake was the dress, with a small doll in the middle. "That's the most beautiful cake I've ever seen," I marveled, walking about it.

The housemother smiled at me. "It was made by a lady who attends your church. She makes a cake for each of the children on their birthday. I'm sure you've seen Mrs. Chapman's cakes before."

Of course I had, but she didn't fix anything half so

elaborate for the church dinners. I had to see if she would make a cake for Kathy's birthday.

When Mrs. Chapman came to the door, she seemed happy to have a visitor. I felt ashamed not to have found time for a visit before. She had me come to her kitchen while she finished a cake. What luck! "I saw a cake you made and was wondering if you'd make one for my daughter's birthday." When she hesitated, I added, "Of course, I'll pay for it."

"I'll draw you the instructions, but I don't make cakes for children who have a mother."

"I'm not very good at things like that," I said.

She smiled. "I wasn't when I started. You know, dear, when children are small any cake made by their mother is beautiful, especially if it was made for them. There's a photograph album in the dining room. Look at it and maybe you'll understand."

As I looked through the album, I could almost feel the excitement of each child's special day. "It's hard to find time for everything," I said, with a feeling of guilt.

"Yes, it was then, too," said Mrs. Chapman. "But we can always find time for the important things. My children thought their cake was the most important part of a birthday. I made it a big project some years to make up for the lack of presents. It was hard to find the time with farm chores and gardening. Now I like to make sure other children have a birthday cake. But I don't make them if their mother can, because I would be taking something special from her."

Fascinated, I watched her hands, stiff from arthritis, form roses on a pastry nail. She deftly shaped the petals of frosting into a work of art. Each flower was placed on a tray to refrigerate until she was ready to use them. As she worked, she let me practice making flowers.

"You are an artist," I said. "I'll never get them right."

She smiled at my lopsided roses. "Just remember that every artist was first an amateur."

Eventually, I lost track of Mrs. Chapman, but I was grateful to that wise woman who made me realize how important a child's birthday is—not just the first or second one either, but on through adolescence. She helped me understand that by giving my children fewer material things and more of myself I would raise better adjusted children. From then on I found time to leave my housework and take a look at the world through a child's eyes. A walk in the woods, a trip to see a neighbor's new kittens or to study an ant hill often proved very educational. But Mary thought of me as odd instead of a good mother.

Ronnie started school before he was five, and to him it was a waste of time. Even then, he marched to a different drummer and thought school was a torture prepared just for him. Like a free spirit, he would have been happier roaming the woods with Pal. He liked some parts of school—recess and coming home were best. The parties were fun, but how I dreaded the Valentine party he was looking forward to. Old hurts came back to haunt me as I watched my little son spread valentines across the table.

"Here's my list," he said with an air of importance. "You can help me pick them out."

But my thoughts were fleeing back over the years to a new girl in class, who sat embarrassed as stacks of valentines piled up on every desk except hers. I'd given as many as I could. And each time a monitor came down the aisle, my hopes would rise. But when the big box was empty, so was my desk. A sick feeling started in the pit of my stomach and moved up into my throat. "I don't care," I told myself over and over. But I did.

"Mom, will you print my name for me?" Ronnie's voice pleaded, bringing me back to dread my small son being hurt the same way.

He picked up his pencil and copied his name on the back of each valentine. "I want to give one to everyone in class."

What would he do if there was nothing in the box for him? "Oh, God," I whispered, "don't let him be hurt."

My fears were over when I saw him dash through the yard with a sack under his arm. "Look, Mom, just look at all the good things I got. I saved some for Kathy 'cause I knew she'd feel bad." And for the next hour, they divided and traded valentines.

Spring brought another incident about adoption. The children and I were raking the back lot when an elderly neighbor came over to talk. Ronnie came running up with a pair of clippers. "Do these belong to Daddy?" he asked.

The woman looked from me to my son. "You'd sure never know he's adopted, he looks so much like you."

Ronnie gave me a startled look, then without a word, he turned and ran into the house. "I'm sorry," she said, "I guess I shouldn't have mentioned it."

"No, you shouldn't have!" I shouted, as I picked up Kathy.

We found Ronnie huddled on his bed with Bear. "Why didn't you tell me I wasn't your kid?" he sobbed.

"Son, we told you Daddy adopted you. Didn't you understand?"

He stopped crying and looked at me. "But you told me you were my mother. You lied!"

"That lady doesn't know what happened. I carried you under my heart just like I did Kathy. I'm sorry you think I lied to you." Cupping his tear stained face in my hands, I looked deep into his eyes. "Like it or not young fellow, I'm your mother. You're stuck with me, and come to think of it, I'd like you even if you weren't mine."

"Aw, Mom," he cried, flinging his arms around me. "I love you."

"Enough to help me finish raking the yard?"

Arm in arm, the three of us went back to work. And for then, all thoughts of adoption were filed away in a far corner of our minds.

Work in the yard didn't go fast with us—there were too many new discoveries. Plants were peeking through the earth, birds were inspecting the freshly raked areas and I loved watching eager little minds discovering the wonders of nature.

We all loved the outdoors, and some of our weekends and vacations were spent on short hiking and camping trips. But one summer we decided to splurge and headed for Yellowstone Park. We had traveled all day and Martin and I were tired. As with most children, our two seemed to increase their energy as ours diminished.

Kathy decided to comb my hair, gently making curls and giggling over the results.

"Wow!" Ronnie gasped. "You should see all the grey hair Mom's got."

Martin grumbled, "You know who caused most of them don't you?"

All was quiet in the back seat for a few seconds. Then came Ronnie's reply, "I guess you did Dad. You've known her longer than we have." They both doubled up with laughter.

Tears were misting my eyes as I reached across the seat. Martin's hand touched mine. Words were not necessary. Our children thought of us as a normal family. With a sigh of deep contentment, I left myself in the care of my back seat beauticians, knowing I would look like a mess when they finished.

The second night out we camped in the Tetons on a slope under some tall pines. We were almost asleep when the children sat up in their sleeping bags and whispered, "What's that noise?"

"It's the wind in the trees," I told them. "Listen quietly and it will put you to sleep." They listened to the sighing of the giant limbs over our tent.

"I'll bet it's angels whispering up there," Ron said. And Kathy agreed. That seemed like a good explanation.

The next morning they watched clouds float above the trees. Ron was fascinated by the height of the pines and remarked, "I'll bet some of them go all the way to Heaven." At times like that I would whisper, "Thank you, Lord."

Chapter 4
It Can't Happen to Us

We live in a society that shuns dying. Parents let their children view killing on television, then shy away from answering a child's questions about death. We know it happens to other people in other places—but not to us, not here.

Pal was first to bring the reality of death to our children. They had attached almost human emotions to all pets, and Pal's life-span had been exceptionally long. Ron missed him one day as soon as he came in from school. The search went on for weeks, but eventually they knew he must be dead.

"What happens when we die?" Ronnie asked one night as we were saying prayers.

"Our soul returns to God," I answered.

Tears rolled down his cheeks. "It makes me cry when I think of Pal not having us with him when he died. I'll bet he was sad."

Holding his sobbing little body, I tried to comfort him as Kathy joined the crying session. And I cried with them, sharing the pain of losing a pet. The grief and eventually the acceptance were things we could share.

Some friends gave them another dog, Taffy, and Mary exploded. "Good grief! You were rid of that overgrown mutt. Why don't you get small pets you can replace without all that crying?"

"I wasn't in any hurry to get another one," I said. "But this little dog was offered. How could you replace a pet without them knowing it?"

"You get small pets like fish, birds, or hamsters. If one dies you simply buy a replacement that looks like it. That's what we do. I've spared my child all that grief."

Mary was even more shocked to learn the children were attending a funeral the next week. Martin's grandfather had been ill for some time. Both children had been aware that people die, but there had been no death in our family during their life.

"You surely don't intend to let them view the body?" Mary asked.

"If they want to. Children went to funerals when I was young. I've tried to explain what will happen. What if Martin or I should die and that was the first funeral they attended? Isn't it better to help them face these things and learn that life isn't all good times?" By then I was feeling rather dubious because I could see the shock and disbelief on her face. She left, acting as though I were some kind of sadist. Why, I thought, do I have to know so many experts who make me feel guilty?

Experts, that was the answer. Dr. Spock suggested: "Don't present it [death] as the end of everything." And he didn't say to hide death from them. It occurred to me that maybe that was one reason his book was so helpful.

He didn't assume a know-it-all attitude and credited the reader with at least a little intelligence: "Trust yourself. You know more than you think you do. Don't take too seriously all the neighbors say. Don't be overawed by what the experts say. Don't be afraid to trust your own common sense."

Ronnie and Kathy asked a lot of questions. Why are people crying if Grandpa is with Jesus? Can Grandpa hear us? We tried to answer as best we could. And in a week their minds were filled with thoughts of school.

Kathy started school and, unlike Ron, she loved it. It was easy to see, even at that age, the Butler family had a real brain on their hands. We were amazed at how fast she learned to read advanced books.

Besides homework, they brought home everything from chicken pox to mumps. From home nurse, I graduated to PTA. Next, I started earning my degree in Cub Scouts, then Campfire Girls—while working part-time. There were days when the house resembled a disaster, and I felt like the old lady in the shoe. But we had our special times.

They did their homework each evening on the kitchen table. While I fixed dinner they told me about their joys and troubles of the day. We called it "the listening hour." If it was serious, it went to a higher court—Dad. A lot of problems were solved at that time. Better still, a lot of them were avoided.

Although we attended church on a fairly regular basis, depression would often close over me. I still had a poor opinion of myself. Often a critical remark would send me to the very depths of hell, putting me through a mental self-flagellation.

Other mothers could get their children ready and in church on time. Not me. By the time the first strains of the organ sounded, I was feeling tired and irritated. To keep peace, we sat between the children. And being normal children, they sighed, squirmed and scribbled, as I scowled and wondered if they heard one word the pastor said.

Most of my worries were silly. Accidents usually happened when I wasn't expecting them. Still, we didn't let the children go anywhere without asking or play out after dark. But someone thought of a thing called trick or treat. I would have loved it during my childhood; we had very little candy and it was safe to go out at night. But they came up with this idea when kids got too much candy and crime had increased. It wasn't so bad when the children were small; one of us went along with them while the other stayed home and passed out treats.

"We feel silly with you going with us," Ron said one Halloween. "I'm big enough to look out for both of us."

Martin looked surprised as they left without me. "I didn't think you would give in so easily."

Hurrying to the bedroom, I pulled on a pair of his jeans and a sweat shirt. By the time I padded myself and pulled one of my stockings over my head, even my kids wouldn't recognize me. "I didn't promise them I wouldn't go," I said, leaving by the back door.

During the next hour, I stayed near the group my children were with. Ronnie kept watching me, making sure I didn't get close to Kathy. Just as I was feeling smug, Ronnie decided to ask for help. "Would you call the police? That guy has been following us," he told a man who was handing out candy.

"We'll see about that," the man said, as he started toward me.

Pulling the stocking off wasn't easy. "I'm their mother," I yelled. They agreed to call it a night before their mother was picked up by the police.

The years, filled with more ups than downs, passed too quickly. Ron grew more serious as he entered his teens, but he still retained his place as family clown. On his 13th birthday, he came into the kitchen and hugged me: "Control yourself, dear Lady, you are now the mother of a teen-ager. Have courage!"

Kathy, our little scholar, usually did twice the amount of required homework. We were proud of her, but eventually we had grown to expect it of her. Unfortunately, her teachers did too. I didn't realize how she pushed herself to get high grades. It seemed easy for her.

My family was surprised and proud when I decided to go to school. By the time I'd convinced myself I wouldn't be the oldest student, most of the classes were full. I finally decided on psychology. This proved to be far more than educational.

In a way, I began to understand Mary. But best of all, I could see and understand many of the conflicts between myself and the world. We can't change what we have been. But through our wise teacher, almost everyone in the class could change what they would be in the future.

That was my first experience with a group that could be open—people who could say, "Look, I've been there. You're not alone in your fears. We're all in this together." It hadn't helped me to hear how perfect Mary was. But it did help to hear people tell about some of the really dumb mistakes they had made.

It was often late by the time I finished my work and lessons. But I enjoyed it, and the difference in my attitude was worth the extra effort.

We decided a second car was necessary with my classes and part-time job. On a visit to my parents, Martin mentioned that he was watching for a good used car. I'll sell you mine," Dad said. This shocked us. Dad without a car—I couldn't remember such a thing. He was so determined, he talked us into taking it that day.

Was it premonition that made me stop at the corner and look back? I will always remember the look on Dad's face as he watched Martin drive off in his car.

A few weeks later the telephone jarred me from a deep sleep. It was Mom, telling me they were taking Dad to the hospital. We knew it was serious for Dad to allow such a trip. Traffic was light, and we were there within an hour. But we didn't make it in time. Dad was dead. He'd had heart trouble for years, yet the suddenness and finality of death hadn't touched my family for a long time.

Mom agreed to go home with my brother. We would all meet the next morning for the final arrangements. Within an hour, we were driving back to the city. The children were asleep and the night was silent except for the tires whining on the highway. As I gazed out of the window, we passed a farm where my parents had once lived. "I never really knew him," I said.

Martin's hand reached over and touched mine. "You probably knew him better than you think."

My mind went back over the years, recalling Dad telling about his wretched childhood. He had known little love, and it had left its scars. I have often wondered what fortune would have held for him if he'd had a better beginning. In his own way, he was a genius.

Dad's mind and cars seemed to work in unison. He was a self-taught mechanic, and often the only one in an area back when cars were rare. But Dad's uncontrolled temper worked against him, and greener hills always beckoned.

I also remembered a man who worked late into the night for money to buy firecrackers or Christmas presents. Mom would blink back tears, wondering how she would pay the bills. The bills were always paid—Dad had his pride, too. A pride that I, in my childish greed, sometimes thought stupid.

During my freshman year of high school, we were living on a farm. I'd had surgery the year before that would have wiped us out if I hadn't been accepted in a children's free hospital. Dad finally relented to me being a charity case—it meant my life or his pride.

As I got off the school bus one evening, I saw a man feeding his hogs grapefruit. My mouth watered at the thought of any citrus fruit. They were simply out of our reach financially. "Are they spoiled?" I asked.

"Naw, we get them from relief. None of us like the sour things so we feed 'em to the hogs."

My taste buds worked overtime on the trip home. I had asked all about getting these free things. Imagine having so many grapefruit you would feed them to hogs. My feet fairly flew as I rounded up the cows and headed them toward the barn. I couldn't wait to tell my parents the good news.

"Dad," I yelled above the noise of our fat dog that greeted me with wild yelps. He was fat because he hunted, often providing our meat, too. I finally made Dad hear me. "I've got the best news. You know the people where I catch the bus? Well," I said, feeling important, "they get new clothes, free. You should see the nice dresses their girl wears to school. Almost as nice as anything in the catalog. And they get grapefruit, too. They don't like them so they throw them to the hogs." By then, I had Mom's undivided attention. She loved citrus fruits almost as much as I did.

"Who told you those things are free?" Dad demanded.

"They did. All you have to do is sign up for something called relief." I stopped, petrified at the rage that came over my father's face.

"We have never been on relief, and no child of mine had better ever let me hear that word again. Shame on you!" he yelled, stomping out of the house.

"You hurt his pride, Honey," Mom said, trying to make me understand.

"Pride!" I yelled. "He can have his pride while we depend on wild game to eat. Those people eat better than we ate when Dad had his garage. Where's that pride when you work like a man on this farm? When we lived in town you cleaned people's houses for some lousy change."

"That's enough! Your father does the best he can," Mom said, getting ready to go milk the cows I had brought in. "You get your lessons," she ordered.

Anger at my father, frustration at an unfair world, and Mom's scolding sent me stomping up the stairs. I felt the rickety steps shudder with each stomp. "I hope the stupid house falls down," I shouted at the walls. "I'll show them, I won't leave this room."

Sprawled across the bed, I let my imagination run wild with thoughts of having anything you wanted to eat or wear. What would it be like, I wondered, to have something to wear that was bought new instead of hoping to get someone's cast-off clothing? And what would it be like to walk into a grocery store and pick out any fruit you wanted to eat? My kids would have those things, I vowed, or I'd be first in line at the welfare office. It didn't occur to me Dad was trying to show me I had to work for what I wanted.

My cat had followed me upstairs and I promised him

some cream when I got rich. I whispered into his ear that we would stay in this room until I decided how I'd become rich and make Dad sorry for his stubborn ways.

The cat's loyalty lasted until the smell of frying rabbit drifted up the stairs. And my empty stomach won the battle against my stubborn mind.

Carrying the books that hadn't been opened, I went to the kitchen. Without one word passing between us, Dad and I ran the milk separator, washed it and put the milk in a cold room.

When Dad was mad, he pouted. Mom would try to coax him out of it. And my brothers, before they'd left home, would argue with him. Not me. I was a chip off the old block. When Dad pouted, I ignored him. We had been known to go for weeks without speaking.

Dad's family were people who could not express or show love. But how they could show their tempers. And Dad was simply a product of his environment. I can never remember him saying "I love you" or "I'm sorry." Sadder yet, I can never remember saying those words to him.

My brother and Mom arrived early the next day. We went to pick out the lot and make all the necessary arrangements. I was astounded at the price of death. The lot—the service—all those expenses had never occurred to me.

Dad's funeral was a shock to Ronnie and Kathy. I was grateful that we had not shielded them from death. They knew that night at the hospital he was dead. But the shock didn't come until they touched Dad's hand. Ronnie called me aside later. "Since I'm his only grandson, I feel he would want me to be a pall bearer."

Our son, half-boy, half-man, was making a quick transition into the adult world with all of its huge responsibilities.

A strange thing happened that night. It seemed as if Dad was calling to me in a dream. "Sissie, you've got to listen to me. Tell Martin to check your brother's back steps. If he doesn't, Mama will fall down them and get hurt."

I sat up in bed, waking Martin. He listened to my dream. "Since Mom is staying at your brother's house, maybe I'd better check the steps when we go over tomorrow."

Martin checked the steps. "They are sound," he said, and we dismissed it as one of my many vivid dreams.

My parents had purchased a house in the city just before Dad died. One day Mom started down her back steps and felt them give. She called us and Martin crawled under the porch where he found the steps rotten and ready to collapse. He had checked the wrong house. My parents had purchased the house my brother had lived in for 20 years. Dad would naturally refer to it as my brother's house since he had never lived there.

Just when things seemed to return to normal, Fluffy was killed by a speeding motorist who had deliberately swerved to hit him. "How could anyone be so mean?" Kathy sobbed. That was a question I couldn't answer.

We wrapped Fluffy in one of Martin's old shirts he had loved to curl up on. He joined other pets in a place marked by violets, and I was quite sure I didn't want another cat.

Why should I get another cat? After the novelty wore off they were mostly mine. But that was probably my fault for talking to animals as though they were people.

There has almost always been a cat in my life. When I stopped to talk to a friend a few weeks later and saw the tiny cute kitten she said nobody wanted, I knew where it would end up.

Although the runt of the litter, the grey ball of fur had spunk. She arched her back and hissed at Taffy as soon as I put her down. Someone remarked, "She acts like the Queen of Sheba." And Sheba pranced across the floor, checking out her new domain.

During the next few months, I asked myself how anything so little could be in so many places at once. She would leave the kitchen and climb to the top of the drapes before I could yell. As though Sheba wasn't enough trouble, I doubled it by accident.

We were running late that morning. Kathy had an early dental appointment before school. As we pulled out of the drive, a grey streak followed by three dogs ran in front of the car.

"How did Sheba get out?" I asked, getting out to rescue the hissing cat. Hurriedly, I took the angry cat from a tree and put it in the basement.

After dropping Kathy at school an hour later, I returned to find a happy kitten in Sheba's bed and our angry cat. It took me several minutes to realize why there were two cats in the basement. They looked so much alike it was impossible to tell them apart without looking close.

The new cat was happy with the arrangement. But I did not want another cat. One cat and one dog. Those were my rules. But several days passed and we still had the cat that had now been named Solomon. What else would go with Sheba? I kept hoping the owners would claim him. He'd had a rough life, if the deep scars on his body meant anything.

Sheba and Taffy were beginning to accept him, and he was beginning to act like a little king. Once he got his tummy full a few times, he thought it was time to get finicky. "No way, mister," I told him. "All kings must give in at times, and you'll learn I rule with a heavy hand." Sheba ate with the finesse of a queen, but Sol had to check everything out usually spilling everything. He was short on manners.

About the time I gave up hope of finding his owners, he broke his hip. For the two weeks his hip was in a cast, I was his handmaid. I would take him to the garden for his daily rituals, when he would look at me as if to say, "What are you waiting for slave-girl? Pick me up!" The little beast was enjoying being waited on. He was taking the name Solomon too seriously.

Both cats loved to play house and dolls with Kathy and her friends. Sheba usually consented to being dressed in doll clothes and pushed around in the doll buggy. After Sol's cast came off, he would only allow it as long as the doll's milk bottle was in his mouth. He became Kathy's new Betsy Wetsy doll. When the milk ran out so did Sol, who was often banned from the room for house-wrecking. Kathy's doll furniture was exactly the right size for a game of cat ping pong.

The day Kathy and several friends decided to play wedding, with Sol and Sheba as the bride and groom, brought another era to a close. Sheba was a reluctant bride, but a scratch in the right place could settle her down.

Nothing could induce Sol to stay for the wedding except force—not even the cookies and milk served for refreshments. They had infringed on his dignity and rights of bachelorhood, and he refused to play house again.

Sol turned his time entirely to Ronnie. He was much happier playing marbles, toy soldiers or curled up in his buddie's arms listening to records. The two seemed to communicate without words.

Part II
Ron's Story

Chapter 5
The Beginning of the End

Ron, as he insisted on being called, made waves in my calm sea of security. He straddled a chair one day after school, watching me intently. "Mom, what would you say if I took ROTC* this year?"

"We've never insisted on you taking any particular subject, Son. But . . ." I shook my head to clear away visions that kept popping into my mind. Row after row of soldiers in beds, on crutches, in wheel chairs. I had planned on being a nurse until I worked in an army hospital during the war.

Ron was watching me, his usually smiling face very serious. "I'll probably have to go in the service. It would be better for me to have some idea what branch I want to be in."

*Reserve Officers' Training Corps

"Why don't you think about it? There's so many subjects you'll need."

"I have thought about it. It seems like everyone should do something important. How can a guy who isn't a football or basketball hero ever be remembered? Face it, Mom, I won't be remembered as the most studious kid. If I can help bring honors to my school through ROTC, I'm as important as some guy getting his brains bashed out on a football field. My mind's made up, unless you or Dad say I can't."

"We wouldn't do that unless your grades drop."

He grinned, a dimple creasing his chin. "We have to keep our grades up or no ROTC." On his way out, he picked up a fresh supply of cookies and gave me a hug. "Thanks, Mom." At the door, he hesitated a second. "That wasn't just for the cookies."

Ron looked good in his uniform. Much to our surprise, he worked harder in his other classes. He would never study as hard as Kathy, but there wasn't any jealousy about her grades. "It's a good thing I'm the oldest," he told me. "Can you imagine having to follow that smart kid through school? The teachers would always make a comparison. Sis gets the break. After having me, teachers will sigh with relief when they get her."

Then came the date that made us all wonder if the world had gone insane. President Kennedy was assassinated. All ROTC units held a memorial service and I knew it affected Ron. He stayed in his room for a long time after he came home.

Kathy finished her homework and went to play. I finally knocked on Ron's door. "Son, is something wrong?"

"No, I just wanted to think." I opened the door and offered him some fruit. "I'm not hungry." Then he looked up and I could see tears in his eyes. "He had everything to live for—money, position and pow! his life is snuffed out like a candle. Has the world gone crazy?"

The violent sixties were in full swing, making a blot on the history of the human race.

Ron progressed in ROTC. He was a member of the city championship drill team, first sergeant of his company and a member of the color guard. But he had his sights aimed higher. As color guard commander, he could carry the American flag. "Next year," he promised, "you'll salute the flag with your favorite son carrying it."

Kathy would be in junior high the following year, but she wasn't very excited about it. The little girl in her wanted to stay in the school she had attended since kindergarten. A new school would mean a change in friends and teachers.

Ron attended ROTC training at an army camp that summer. Kathy signed up for a swimming class, determined to be a better swimmer. "Honey," I scolded, "do you have to be best at everything?" She was very nearsighted so I worried about her swimming when Ron wasn't with her.

"It's not that," she said. "I'll never swim like Ron. The kids are calling me fatso and I want to lose weight."

Kathy's weight problem was beginning to be a touchy subject with me. I had been a skinny child and writhed under people's remarks about it. This has to be a normal world, and Heaven help the poor child who doesn't fit the mold. Nothing made me madder than having some overweight adult make a remark about Kathy being fat. Nothing that is, except sly remarks like: "I've heard that sometimes a mother feels guilty if she doesn't love a child and makes up for it by stuffing them with food."

There's no way to make anyone lose weight until they want to. It seemed Kathy was ready, so I went to the park with her.

We had planned on visiting Ron at camp the first Sunday. How we missed him. "I'll bet he's having such a good time he'll forget about us coming," I said one evening. A few minutes later the telephone rang. We heard Martin say, "Son, is anything wrong?" Kathy and I ran to the phone. Ron talked to each of us, saying he just wanted to make sure we hadn't forgotten the visit.

As soon as church was over, we headed for camp. It seemed strange to realize the young soldier coming toward us was Ron. The whole thing looked too real, making me realize our son was growing up. I knew he couldn't stay a child forever. This was too sudden in an uncertain world. Like most mothers, I worried about him driving in a few months. Vietnam was a rumble in the distance that also worried me. Watching Ron acting more like a soldier than a teen-ager only emphasized the reality of war. An uneasy feeling stayed with me.

Something else bothered me that day. All of the parents had been invited, but few came. Although the boys tried to hide it, the disappointment was there. "It's baseball season," Ron said. "Some of the guys were betting their dads wouldn't miss a game to come."

Ron seemed reluctant for the day to end. Each time we started to leave, he thought of something else to show us. By the time we drove away, leaving him standing with a group of his buddies, my tears were flowing. Kathy was waving out the rear window. "Ronnie didn't want us to leave," she said. "Why did he act so sad?"

"I guess he was homesick. Remember the time we left you at Grandma's and had to come get you two days later?"

"But I was little and Ronnie's a big kid."

Her description of her brother broke the sad spell. That's true of adults, I thought. We are just big kids, and homesickness doesn't have any respect for age.

The following Wednesday Ron called. "Mom, I'm at the bus station. Could you come get me?"

I hadn't had time to ask why he came home early. My mind thought of a thousand reasons as I drove through the heavy traffic. Ron was waiting on the corner as I drove up. He threw his gear into the back seat and slid in beside me. "I feel rotten. They wanted to take me to the base hospital."

"How long have you felt like this?" I asked, feeling his head. "There's no fever."

"I'm not really sick. That's why I wouldn't go to the hospital. I just feel bad."

He said very little on the way home. I tried not to pry, wondering if there had been some other reason for his sudden return. That is one of the hard problems facing a parent—when to talk and when to keep quiet. If you ask too many questions you're prying. If you don't ask enough, you don't care.

Ron went to his room and didn't wake up until Martin came home. They talked for a few minutes, then Ron called, "Hey, Mom, what's to eat? Your son is starving." That sounded normal.

He straddled a chair and watched me finish the meal. "Sorry I was such a dud this morning. I feel great now. If it wasn't for them thinking I was some kind of a nut, I'd go back. Anyway, my foot hurts a little."

"You didn't mention anything about your foot."

"I'd almost forgotten it. One of the guys hit me on the foot with a canteen. I've never had anything that light hurt so bad. It's still sore."

The soreness was gone the next day. Ron decided against returning to camp. Our vacation was the next week, and he could get the camping gear ready.

Even then, I think something inside was telling me to enjoy this particular time of life, to grasp each moment and hold on because it would never come again.

At the last minute we changed our plans to drive to Florida when Ron asked if we could return to the Ozarks. It didn't make any difference to the rest of us. It was an extremely hot summer and the long drive wasn't very appealing.

The campgrounds were crowded with people trying to escape the city heat. Ron had brought his scuba gear, so we didn't expect him to check in except for meals.

Within an hour, he was back. He dropped the wet gear and flopped on the ground. I went over and knelt beside him. "Is something wrong?"

He sat up, shaking his head. "I don't know. I'm sort of dizzy. You know, now that I think of it, that's how it started at camp."

"Do you want to go home?"

"It's probably the heat. I should have known better than dive in the cold water after racing Kathy to the river."

Martin returned to camp and we were trying to decide whether to leave or wait until morning. "Oh, forget it!" Ron said. "I'm not sick. It's growing pains."

But he didn't have enough pep to keep up with Kathy for the next two days. On the third day we headed home. Kathy didn't mind. She was lonesome for her pets, and Ron's quiet spells seemed to affect us all.

I made an appointment with the doctor as soon as we reached home. Ron grumbled about wasting time and money. The doctor checked him over, looked at the foot, then agreed with Ron. "Nothing wrong with this guy except growing pains. He's grown a lot in the past year. I wish all my patients were half as healthy as him."

In a few days, Ron returned to being a normal teenager—reminding us he could start driving soon, talking about the future, what a mess the world was in, and teasing his sister.

Chapter 6
A Time to Laugh, a Time to Cry

It's strange how the memory of one particular day will linger for years. I remember one vivid fall day that looked as though the Master Painter had just finished a great work of art. Never, at any time in my life, had I felt so much at peace with the world. Yet my future had never been more clouded. But on that day, life seemed wonderful.

It seemed unbelievable that Kathy, at 13, was in junior high and Ron, almost 16, was a junior in high school. I was the mother of two teen-agers.

The fruits, the results of our training, would soon start showing up. Nearly 3,000 years ago, one of the wisest men who ever lived told parents: "Train up a child in the way he should go: and when he is old, he will not depart from it" (Proverbs 22:6).

We had tried. But I had seen many kids turn out different than their parents raised them. And the first four years of the sixties should have been enough to scare most of us out of our security blankets. But not on that day. Life was too good to borrow trouble.

I mentally thanked God for all the little everyday things I took for granted. Then school let out and I thanked Him for the two teens racing for the front seat. Ron won, and Kathy pouted in the back seat until one of Ron's friends asked if he could ride. He got in back, and Kathy made sure her friends saw him.

Ron started staying after school to practice drilling. He was determined to carry our flag. Kathy was being a problem. The students were separated according to their grades. She was in a class of high achievers. The strain of trying to make the best grades was telling on her. It was a session of tears almost every night.

Ron made color guard commander, and I thought maybe we were making too much of it. I tried to give Kathy more time and attention. But what she wanted, I couldn't give her—to be at the top of her class.

The next two months were filled with sessions with her teachers. What possessed her to drive herself was beyond me. While I often wished Ron's attitude about his grades was different, I felt Kathy's was wrong, too. There seemed to be no happy medium.

Her counselor called me in for a conference. I got there early and squirmed on the chair wondering if all the teachers thought we beat our child to make her get good grades. Visiting school always seemed to transform me into a self-doubting child again. By the time the counselor came in, I was feeling as if I'd failed somewhere. But she soon put me at ease and we talked about Kathy's drive to be tops.

"Is there no in between?" I blurted out. "Our son is happy to pass and Kathy must be at the top or it's a major crisis."

"I'll talk to her," she promised. "We'll work it out. I wanted to make sure you were aware of her problem."

Another worry was added to the list one evening when they were doing homework. Ron turned to get up and hit his foot on the table leg. He moaned and grabbed his foot.

I picked up the books he dropped. "You didn't hit the table that hard, Son," I said, jokingly. "It's not going to get you out of homework."

He looked up with tears in his eyes. "This is for real, Mom. It still hurts and it looks funny."

There was a small hard lump on the bottom of his foot. "We're going to the doctor tomorrow. I don't like the way this looks."

"This is the same foot that hurt me so bad at camp—remember? I told you how it hurt when the canteen hit it. That's the way it hurt just now. Only I didn't have this lump, then.

The doctor looked at the foot and sent us to a laboratory for some tests. When the tests came back, he seemed more puzzled than ever. "I'm going to send you to a specialist," he said. "We'll see if he can figure out what it is." The first appointment the specialist had open was three weeks away.

Then, as though we didn't have enough worries, Martin's company was put up for sale. It was hard to get into the spirit of the approaching holidays.

On the day of Ron's appointment, I had a bad case of nerves. Sometimes the unknown can scare you, and I was afraid to even think about the word cancer. I knew very little about it. There had never been any in our family. I kept telling myself that a person as healthy looking as Ron couldn't have anything very serious.

The specialist didn't spend ten minutes with Ron. He told me to call the next day about the X-rays.

We left in high spirits. The doctor seemed to think it was just a bruise. And the next day the report was even better. The X-rays didn't show a thing.

Things were looking up. Besides the good news about Ron, Kathy seemed to be making a better adjustment. Although they were teen-agers, Christmas still brought all the magic and traditions they had helped make. We had turkey for Jesus' birthday with the rest of it for Ron's—and there was a cake for each day. Nothing had changed much except the presents. Where there once had been a list of toys, there was now a list of clothes.

I worked late on Christmas Eve and stopped by to pick up Mom. The house had been cleaned for the holidays and I'd left specific orders that it had better stay that way. When we came in, I was horrified to see a stomach churning mess on the floor and Sheba beside it.

"Looks like Sheba upchucked her dinner," Ron said.

"Have you run out of paper towels," I asked, glaring at my family. "Good grief! Couldn't one of you clean this up?"

Grabbing a handful of towels and shoving the cat back, I started cleaning up the mess. Something like that made me sick. Martin knew it, yet he stood there with a silly grin on his face.

Angry at my apparently daffy family, embarrassed that Mom had witnessed this ridiculous scene, and about to vomit myself, I wadded up the towels. It wouldn't give, so I rolled the towels tighter. The mess plopped out on the floor, the cat pounced on it, and both kids howled with laughter. Martin retained his laughter until he knew what my reaction was going to be.

"Daddy took us shopping and I got it for Ron's

Christmas present. Isn't it neat?" Kathy asked.

I picked up the piece of plastic that looked real enough to make me gag. "That is about the most repulsive thing I've ever seen for a present!"

"Aw, Mom," Ron scolded, "it's real cool. Think of the fun I'll have at school."

Kathy giggled. "He's a poet and doesn't know it."

It was easy to forgive them when I recovered from my shock and found a nice meal waiting. The three of them had worked hard to fix dinner and prepare things ahead to help me for the next day.

All of us attended communion service that night. It put us in a receptive mood for our favorite day of the year. It was our custom to open presents on Christmas Eve, because some guest would be sure to arrive early the next morning.

On the morning of Ron's 16th birthday, I let him sleep late. Kathy and I were working a puzzle when he joined us. "What kind of cake do you want?" I asked.

He made a big production of deciding on chocolate. "Since it's my cake, how about me decorating it?"

"Oh, no," Kathy groaned. "I can see what you'll do to it."

But it was his cake, and a few hours later I turned him loose with a big batch of icing. Knowing him, I had doubled the recipe. More would go in the boy than on the cake.

He was proud of his work, and we had to admit it wasn't too bad. I had asked him if he wanted to have a small party. But he didn't seem interested in having even his close friends over.

After dinner he opened his presents, played a few games with Kathy and went to his room. When I went in to kiss him goodnight, he was almost asleep.

"Don't you feel well, Ron?"

"Oh, sure . . . just tired. I guess old age is catching up to me."

He was listless during the next week of vacation. I called the doctor and he said there was a lot of flu. "Give him a lot of fluid and let him rest," he said.

Although Ron insisted on going back to school, I knew he didn't feel well. He thought it was too important to miss. "Aw, Mom, I've worked so hard for color guard. If I miss, it'll put us behind."

It seemed to me they were practicing too hard when he went to bed earlier every night. I couldn't believe the sleep he required, yet it was harder to get him up each morning.

When I left work Christmas Eve, I had told them I wouldn't be back for a few months. Two classes a week were keeping me busy. Studies didn't come easy after all my years away from school.

In February, Ron was to be in a program at Kathy's school. "Wow!" she yelled. "Wait 'till I tell the kids the guy carrying the American flag is my brother." Ron blushed and loved every word.

Parents hadn't been invited, but I went. The color guard performed beautifully. My heart swelled with pride as I watched my son, standing so tall and proud, holding the flag. A lump came in my throat and I remembered a small Cub Scout asking, "Daddy, what is that funny feeling I get in my throat when the flag is raised?"

His daddy put his arm around the boy's shoulder and replied, "That's called patriotism, Son, or maybe just pride in Old Glory."

Ron looked up at his dad. "It's kind of a nice feeling, huh?"

The program was over and the color guard marched smartly through the gymnasium. They fixed the flags and Ron asked one of the fellows to take them to their school. "Sure thing, Ron," the boy said. "I hope you feel better Monday."

Ron slumped on a bench, his face ashen. "Mom, my foot hurts so much I can hardly stand it," he said, unlacing his combat boot. "Look!" he gasped.

I looked and tried not to panic. The foot was all puffy. As soon as Kathy came out we headed for the doctor's office. He called the specialist and made an appointment for the next day. From his side of the conversation, we knew the other doctor wasn't happy about an extra patient on Saturday. The doctor gave Ron something for pain and said to soak the foot in hot water.

The medicine made him sleepy and he went to bed early. There was little sleep for me that night. Each time I'd hear a noise, I'd go check Ron. He seemed to be resting. But an uneasy feeling was gnawing at me. Something was wrong. Sitting by his bed that night, I made up my mind that they were not going to put us off again. They had said, "Wait until school is out. If it hasn't gone away by then, we'll put him in the hospital for tests."

The specialist looked at the foot and made arrangements for Ron to enter the hospital in two days. There weren't the complaints I had expected. In fact, Ron seemed rather quiet. The morning he left for the hospital, he stood, suitcase in hand, looking at his room.

"Did you forget something, Son?"

He gave a deep sigh. "Have you ever had a premonition, Mom? I had it just now. As I turned to look at my room, I had the feeling that nothing will ever be the same again."

Yes, I knew what he meant. A feeling of sadness had

been with me for several days, but I couldn't tell him that. "Everyone has qualms about the hospital."

"I guess so," he said. "Let's go."

Once Ron was entered, they started routine tests to prepare him for surgery. It had been decided our family doctor would assist the specialist. Before I left, Ron called me back. "Mom, under no circumstances are you to let them take my leg off."

My knees gave way and I slumped into a chair. "Son," I gasped, "there's been no mention of such a thing."

"Promise me," he urged.

"I can't. What if it meant your life?"

"There's a lump on my ribs and one on my shoulder. See," he said, holding his shirt up.

"When did you notice these?"

"This morning. Amputating my leg wouldn't help. I'll tell the doctor about these lumps. There might not be any connection. But I don't want one of those guys taking away my future in the operating room."

It was a good thing we lived close to the hospital. I was in no condition to drive. By the time I talked to the doctor, Ron had called him. "We'll just wait and see," he said. After I told Martin and Kathy about the new lumps, dinner was only picked at. Time seemed to drag until visiting hours.

Ron was propped up in bed, angry as a hornet. "Do you realize I'm on the children's floor? Everyone under 18 is considered a child. Wow!" he said, waving his hands. "Can't you just hear the guys at school when they come to visit me in the kids ward?"

"Calm down," Martin told him. "The doctor said you would only be here two or three days."

Just then a pretty aide brought him some juice.

"Ron!" she squealed. "I didn't know you were here. Wait till I tell the other girls. We'll all come visit you."

"Well," he said, after she left, "this floor may have its good points at that." Before visiting hours were over, several aides had stopped by.

The operation was scheduled for eight the next morning. But a strange feeling came over me as I was fixing breakfast. Martin had taken the day off, but it was decided that Kathy would go to school. At least school would keep her busy. The feeling persisted and I decided to leave for the hospital right then. Martin said he would take Kathy to school, then join me.

I felt something was wrong as I hurried into the hospital. When the elevator door opened, I heard Ron's slurred voice. "No . . . not leaving . . . my parents aren't here . . . not leaving."

His hands were pushing at two attendants who were trying to move him through the door.

"Where are you taking him?" I asked.

"To surgery," one answered. "They want him now. He's already had his medication."

"Mom," Ron called. "Mom, is that you?" He could hardly open his eyes as I reached down and kissed him. "How did you know to come early?"

"I felt you needed me. Do you want me to go down on the elevator with you?"

"Didn't want to go without telling you . . . Dad . . . Kathy . . . how much I love you . . . Mom, are you still here?" he said, when they wheeled him into the elevator.

"Yes, I'm still with you. I'll go with you as far as I can."

"Did you pray? I did . . . Everything's going to be fine."

"This is as far as you can go," the attendant said. "You can wait in that room."

"Son, I'll have to leave you here. I love you," I whispered in his ear.

He tried to smile. "I love you, too. Don't worry, I'm in good hands."

Tears blinded me as I slumped on a couch in the waiting room. The room was empty, so I allowed myself the luxury of a good cry before I called Martin. He was angry because the hospital hadn't told us about the change. By the time he arrived, the room had begun to fill up. A volunteer passed out coffee and everyone settled down to wait.

No matter how many people are there, a hospital waiting room is a sad, lonely place. Each one is lost in his thoughts and prayers for the loved one down the hall. I read magazines, studied the cracks in the ceiling, and mentally wandered back through good memories. It seemed as though we had waited an eternity.

"Something has gone wrong," I whispered to Martin. "It's been four hours. The doctor said two hours at the most."

"Don't borrow trouble, Honey. Remember when Kathy had her tonsils out? The schedule was mixed up and they forgot to tell us."

For the past hour, I had noticed the difference in the way doctors told the family about the patient. If they came into the room all smiles—everything was fine. But if they called the family out in the hall, the news was bad. A few cried, some left, while others just sat staring at the floor. I started to mention it, as our doctors motioned for us to come into the hall.

"I'm afraid we have bad news," our family doctor said. "It's cancer. We also checked the other tumors.

It's highly metastasized. I'm sorry."

Rage surged over me until I thought I would choke. For months they had said it was nothing. Now they were sorry. Just as I was about to tell them my thoughts, I felt Martin slump toward the floor. We caught and held him.

"Do you want some medication?" a doctor asked.

Martin shook his head. "What about Ron? What kind of treatment can they give him?"

"That will depend on what the lab comes up with. We will know in a few days. You go back in the waiting room. Ron just went to recovery so it'll be some time before you can see him." And both doctors hurried away, anxious to escape the wrath I'm sure they could see on my face.

We held each other. "Honey, what are we going to do?" Martin sobbed. "We can't lose him. Oh, God," he moaned, "why him?"

"Dear Jesus," I whispered, "we've never needed You more than now."

Chapter 7
A Sign of Hope

Mom's minister brought her to the hospital as soon as we called, but it was late afternoon before Ron recognized anyone. "Grandma, what are you doing here?" he asked. "I'm not that bad, am I?"

"I just wanted to see if you needed anything," Mom told him, trying to keep the anguish from her voice. But he felt too bad to talk and drifted back and forth in a painful haze.

Martin looked as though he would drop. I talked him into going home and coming back later with Kathy. After everyone left, Mom and I sat beside Ron—waiting. Thousands of questions swirled through my mind, also anger at the doctors for not being more alert and at myself for not calling in another doctor.

An arm went around my shoulders. "Mom," Kathy whispered, "is Ron asleep?" I nodded, watching her worried face for any sign that Martin had told her.

After a few minutes, Martin insisted it was time for me to go home. "Take Kathy with you," he said. "I'll stay until visiting hours are over."

Kathy fixed me something to eat and pulled her chair close to me. "What did the doctors say? I know it's bad because Daddy couldn't talk about it."

How much, Lord? How much shall I tell her? "Do you know what cancer is?"

"Yes, we studied it in health."

"Ron has some type of cancer. They haven't told us what kind."

Tears rolled down her cheeks. "It said in the book there is no cure for it."

"Your book is at least two years old, Honey. They are getting new medicine all the time."

She ran into her room and I could hear her crying, then praying.

When Martin and Mom came in, they said Ron had complained about being sore. A doctor said they'd had a little trouble during surgery. What kind of trouble? Had his heart stopped? We never knew. It seemed we were expected to pay medical bills and get little information.

During the next week both doctors made themselves scarce. We couldn't reach them at all and they gave no information to Ron. On Saturday, I called the specialist. His nurse started telling me why he could not talk right then. "If I don't talk to the doctor today, don't bother sending me a bill."

The doctor returned my call shortly. "I'm sorry," he said. "We should have talked to you several days ago. The tests show lymphosarcoma. It's . . . almost always fatal."

My mind wouldn't accept what he was saying. "Are

you telling me there's no hope?"

"Yes, your doctor will make him as comfortable as possible. Are you there alone?"

"My husband and daughter are here."

"Good, I do have to get back to my patients. I'm very sorry," he said, and hung up.

"No!" I sobbed, dropping the telephone. "They are wrong!" Martin and Kathy ran to me and I told them what I'd just heard. The three of us clung together for strength and cried ourselves out.

Ron's spirits improved when he was allowed visitors. Flowers lined his wall, stacks of cards were stuffed in his closet and as soon as school was out each day, the visitors started. Except for the pain, he was loving all the attention. I had gotten in the habit of going to visit each morning. He ordered coffee and played host to me.

One morning gave us a forewarning of the hurt feelings, confusion, and grief that was to follow. Kathy was getting an award and Ron urged me to go. Before I could get dressed, I'd had five calls. I was frantic as it neared time for the program to begin. Before I got out the door, the phone rang again. It could be the hospital, I thought. But it was a relative. "Please," I begged, near tears, "I don't have time to talk."

"Is Ron worse?"

"No, I'll call you later. I've got to hurry." My voice broke and I hung up.

The program had started when I arrived. Kathy's teacher had saved a place for me. She reached over and placed her hand on mine. That gentle squeeze said so much.

After the program, Kathy gave me her certificate to show Ron. I hurried to the hospital and found him waiting when I got off the elevator. "Mom, what happened this morning? Dad called here to see if I was sick. He said for you to call him."

We found a phone and called Martin. "Honey, what was wrong this morning? After I talked to Ron, I thought you or Kathy had been hurt. What's going on?"

"Nothing except a lot of calls that made me late for the program. You know I cry when I'm mad."

"By the time it got to Mom, you were crying because Ron was worse. Mom called me at work so I was frantic. We're going to put a stop to this."

After that incident Ron and I decided on a system. Each side of the family would get information from our mothers. Church members would check with the minister. "And that will leave the line clear for my friends to keep me up on school news," Ron added.

When I left, he got in his wheelchair and went to the elevator with me. "Get some rest this afternoon, Mom. You look beat!" He was being kind. I looked horrible.

This was the beginning of a time in Ron's life when he would change the ways of many people. He didn't do it intentionally. I'm sure he wasn't aware how the Lord was working through him to reach others. One such incident happened that day.

Jenny, expecting her second baby, came to visit Ron. They were chattering away, when I stopped by after picking up Kathy. Jenny discovered she was out of cigarettes. "Can I get anything for any of you?" she asked.

"Get me a couple packs of cigarettes," Ron said.

That startled me as much as it did her. "You shouldn't smoke!" she gasped.

"Why not? Am I too young? I'm older than that baby you're expecting. If your smoking won't hurt it, why would it hurt me?"

Jenny looked at Ron, her face flushing. "You made

your point. I'll quit." To my knowledge she never smoked again.

The doctor released Ron after two weeks, with orders to use a wheelchair or crutches. We picked up a very happy patient.

"Home at last!" he shouted, hobbling into his room. "Hi room, did you miss me?"

Martin put the wheelchair beside the bed. "Son, if your room answers back, I'm leaving."

"Dad," he said, grabbing at the cats. "You don't know how good it is to be home."

The next day I started to change the dressing on Ron's foot. "They haven't taken the stitches out," I gasped. "Did they say why?"

"I thought they were the kind that dissolved."

An angry doctor came an hour later to take out the stitches someone had forgotten. The foot was twice the normal size and medicine didn't ease the pain. Removing the stitches hurt so bad he would let Ron rest before going on.

When we went to the doctor a week later, the foot was still larger. We were out of the office in five minutes with a prescription for pain pills.

Meanwhile, the school had installed a home teaching device in Ron's room. He could listen in and take part in two classes. "Ron, are you with us?" they would ask. I took his papers to the teachers and they gave me extra assignments to help him pass that semester.

I wrote to a medical center for information concerning treatment for Ron. Maybe the doctors were going to give up, but I wasn't. The medical center said they would contact our doctor and tell him about the treatment they used. At the same time, newspapers carried an article about a new breakthrough in cancer treatment by a hospital in the East. I sent a letter, giving the details I had copied from the insurance forms. By return mail, we received bad news. They had nothing that would work on lymphosarcoma. This sort of news release is cruel. It gives false hope when, in reality, they had nothing local hospitals didn't have.

On Kathy's birthday, some of the family came for a party. Her aunt brought her a cake that looked like one of the Beatles and a Beatle wig. We gathered at the table and Ron couldn't resist putting on a show. He put the wig on and did a good imitation of the latest Beatle record. For a time, we forgot the wheelchair and why Ron was in it.

A bad case of flu kept Kathy and me home from the Easter service. Martin had to be nurse to all of us.

After church the minister came by with a large pot of Easter lilies for Ron. Before the day was over, he had three sent from other churches.

"When the blooms go off, I want you to plant them outside my window. That way, I can see them bloom next spring."

The pain pills were not easing the foot at all. He was wild with pain when I went to the drug store for another bottle. "Are you sure those are the right thing?" I asked the druggist. "They don't seem to help."

He checked and asked what type of pain they were for. I explained about the operation. "These things are about like taking aspirins. Your son needs something stronger. Get that doctor for me."

The doctor wasn't in, and I tried again when I got home. I called from the extension in the basement. "Ron needs something stronger for pain," I told him. "The druggist said this wasn't strong enough to help."

"Ron will have to learn to live with it. You don't seem to understand. He might live three months. What do you want—a drug addict?"

"What do you mean by three months?" I gasped. "The Medical Center said they were sending you their method of treatment."

"The medicine they recommended is very expensive. You people don't have that kind of money. And for what? One month, maybe two extra ones?"

"Won't you try? At least give him something a little stronger for pain," I begged.

"No," he said curtly.

"Then I'll find a doctor who will," I sobbed, banging down the receiver.

"Mom, are you OK?" Ron asked from the stairs.

"How long have you been standing there?"

He came over and put his arms around me. "It's OK. I've known all along. Don't cry." Ron awkwardly patted my shoulder, then took my hands in his.

"You've known what all along?" I asked.

"That they found cancer and there isn't much hope for my future."

"Ron, there is a treatment. They don't claim it's a cure, just that it prolongs the disease. Sometimes it causes a remission."

He picked the cat up and stroked her head. "In other words, we buy time—hoping for a cure to turn up. What about the cost?"

"They haven't told me. Our insurance would pay part of it. Who told you there was no hope?"

"Do you remember how I met you at the elevator after I could use the wheelchair? One day I was there watching out the window for you. People waiting for the elevators couldn't see me. A nurse from my floor was talking to another nurse. They mentioned the teen-age boy who had terminal cancer.

"You know, there I was sitting there feeling sorry as all get out for the guy. I went back to my room to get a book, because I realized it wasn't time for you. A lady was changing my bed, and I asked her how many teenagers were on the floor. She said, 'You're the only one we've got, Ron. That's why we're spoiling you.'

"Mom, I didn't believe it then. Now I don't know. If this pain doesn't let up, I'd just as soon die. But I'll do what I can. There's $300 in my savings."

For a few minutes, I held him close and enjoyed the sheer delight of loving him. "That money is for your car, remember?"

He held his foot out in front of him. "That thing doesn't make me feel like driving. I thought I'd mess around with my lathe. Maybe it'll take my mind off my foot."

I turned the lights on in his workshop and pulled a stool near his lathe. "Try to stay off your feet. I'll go fix dinner."

He nodded, already lost in thought about his next wood project. I hurried upstairs, not only to start dinner, but to make another call. I needed advice from a doctor, and Martin's company doctor was the only one I could think of.

Dr. Edwards listened as I explained what had happened. "I don't even know what lymphosarcoma is," I said, trying to control my shaking hands.

"It's a malignant disease of lymphatic tissue. Clinically, it's similar to Hodgkin's disease. The diagnosis has to be made by a biopsy."

"Would another doctor take the case? Or would they all refuse to give him something for pain?" I had lost control of myself completely and almost dropped the phone.

"There is an internist working with me. Would you want him to take the case?"

"I'm sorry, Doctor," I sobbed. "I don't know what an internist is."

"He specializes in internal medicine. Listen, you sound as though you need a doctor. Can you bring the boy to my office tomorrow? Both of us will be here. We'll take a biopsy and send it to a different lab. Meanwhile, I'll check with the Medical Center. Have your druggist call me. I'll send something for pain and something to calm you. Both of you get a good night's sleep."

When I called the druggist, he promised to send the medicine right away. Then I prayed. "Please, God, let it ease Ron's pain. Help us!"

I could hear the lathe whining, and my mind could picture Ron's long, slender fingers holding a piece of wood that he would turn into a work of art. He was proud of his woodworking tools and the fact he had bought most of them. The shrill sound of the lathe made me wonder if that was the way Ron was screaming inside.

True to his word, the druggist sent the medicine within an hour. I asked the delivery man to step in while I paid him. "How's the boy?" he asked.

When I looked surprised, he added, "My boy goes to school with him. Said he heard Ron had something wrong with his foot. Hope it's nothing serious."

"We won't know until more tests are made," I said, hoping the word "cancer" didn't spread like wild-fire through the school.

I took one of the pills and a glass of water to Ron. He turned the lathe off as I went in. "I have something for your pain."

He swallowed the pill without question, then reached for his crutches. When we got to the steps, he handed me the crutches and crawled up the steps like a baby.

"This is a lot faster," he called over his shoulder. He collapsed on a chair. "Now," he said, a big grin spreading over his face, "tell me what you threatened to do to the doctor."

"I called Dr. Edwards. He wants me to bring you to his office tomorrow."

"Did he prescribe the pills?"

"Yes, he said there was no reason for you to suffer like that. If the pain is eased off, you may get some rest tonight."

He sat looking wistfully out the window, watching Kathy and half the neighborhood playing on the swings. One of the boys saw Ron watching and waved. Ron waved back, still liking the way younger boys looked up to him. "Isn't it weird? If I could, I wouldn't think of going out there with that silly bunch of kids. But now, because I can't, I want to go out and race around like them."

"Are you forgetting you're only three years older than those silly kids?"

Pulling himself up on his crutches, he took one last look out the window. "I feel like an old man—a tired old man who needs a rest. I'll go lay down and listen to records."

By the time dinner was ready, Ron's pain had eased. He ate a good meal and got a good night's rest.

The next morning we were at the doctor's office early. Dr. Edwards examined Ron and under local anesthetic removed a small tumor the size of a pea from Ron's chest.

"We'll send this in for a biopsy. People have made mistakes on these reports. Let's hope this is one of those times."

"And if it isn't?" Ron asked.

"Then we'll check with different medical centers for the best treatment."

Dr. Edwards introduced us to the internist, Dr. Jordon, who seemed to take an instant liking to Ron. They talked in the outer office while we waited for a sudden shower to stop.

The rain stopped as suddenly as it had started. And I pulled out of the parking lot full of hopes for the future. We had just crested the hill when Ron asked me to pull out of the traffic. "Look," he said, as I stopped. "A rainbow, God's sign of hope."

A beautiful rainbow arched across the sky like a pathway to Heaven. "Do you want to go look for the pot of gold at the end?" I asked.

"Maybe there isn't a pot of gold. Maybe that's where Heaven is." He sat watching the rainbow fade. "Scientists could give you a logical explanation for a rainbow. But I like to think God uses it to let us know He's still with us."

"You know," I said, hugging him, "you're a very philosophical young man. I think I'd like you even if you weren't my son."

"That works the other way, too," he answered.

I started the car and headed home, feeling that maybe there was some hope.

Chapter 8
Buying Time

Happiness can have a short life. It can end with a lab report and a telephone call. We'd had two days of hope when the doctor called. "We want Ron to enter the hospital for more tests," he said.

"Have you heard from the lab?" I asked, fearing the answer.

"Yes, it was the same. The X-rays show some tumors in the lungs. We want to start chemotherapy on him. But we need to know how far the disease has progressed and how much damage has been done. Talk to him. Explain that it isn't going to be easy. We don't know what results we'll have. But I do want to warn him—he'll be very sick before he gets any better. It reacts differently on each individual. If he can't take it, we'll look for another treatment."

"There's something else," he said. "Please don't have any visitors who can't control their emotions. He's going to get depressed and upset without others making it worse. I'll have my nurse call you after she checks the hospital."

Ron looked up when I went to his door. He was listening to his English class. The teacher asked him a question. He answered, then smiled at me, proud he'd been right.

Not now, I thought, let him have this at least. I pulled up a chair and listened to the class discussion. He enjoyed the classes, and a hospital stay would put him behind. The teacher gave Ron his assignment, then told him good-bye. He marked his lesson in his book, then looked up. "Who called?"

"They want you to go in the hospital. It'll be a different one this time."

"Is it necessary?" he groaned. "I feel better now. Besides, I'll get behind on these two classes. It cost a lot of money to install this thing for me."

It isn't easy explaining to a teen-ager why the hospital is more important than school. It isn't easy to explain why a disease can suddenly turn your life upside down. But he tried to understand and agreed to go.

The nurse called and said to take him to the hospital that afternoon. Panic washed over me. I hadn't expected it so soon.

Ron packed his bag, told the pets good-bye, and pulled himself up on his crutches. "Here I go again," he sighed. At the door he turned back for a last look at his things. Sheba was sitting on his desk watching. "Take care of my room," he told her, "and don't go knocking everything off."

We hadn't much more than got him to the room, when X-ray sent for him. The nurse helped him put on pajamas, while I put his things away. "He's scheduled for tests all afternoon," she said. "If you live near, you may as well go home."

The house seemed so quiet without a radio or records playing. The emptiness—the aloneness—closed in on me. I knew I should call our families. But not just yet. There would be questions I couldn't answer. At times I felt as though the questions, the unasked-for advice, and guesses would shove me over the edge.

Martin and Kathy came home and made the calls for me. We ate in silence, each asking, "Why us, Lord?"

We decided to divide the visiting hours instead of all going at once. Martin went that evening and reported Ron was in high spirits.

They started the injections the next morning. On the second day, Ron was very ill and the depression started. "Do you know why they put me in a room with older men?"

"It's all they had open, Son. We'll move you when they have something else."

"No, that's not it. The doctor said he wanted me to see that other people are suffering. Well, they aren't 16. What have I got to look forward to? I'm not going to let them experiment on me . . . stick needles in me." Tears were running down his face. I wiped them away, trying to control myself.

The doctor came in then. He sat down and talked to Ron. I stumbled into a nearby lounge and cried. A nurse followed me in. "It's the medicine," she explained. "When they first start it, they get deeply depressed. It goes away. He misunderstood what the doctor said."

When I calmed down, I returned to Ron's room. Dr. Jordon had calmed him, too. "I'm sorry, Mom. I didn't mean to act like such a baby." He took my hand and kissed the palm, then curled my fingers over it. "Hold on to that and remember I love you."

It seemed as though I spent a lot of time praying those next two weeks. A lot of other people were also praying for Ron. His blood count had dropped so low, it was dangerous to continue the treatment. He came home. My job was to build his blood up so they could start the injections again. The nausea was gone in a few days and he started eating everything I fixed.

Once he was home, his depression left. He was behind in his studies, but he worked hard to catch up. I took his assignments to school. Some of the teachers worked hard to help him pass that year and others couldn't have cared less. It was the same with the students. Most of the kids cared, but occasionally I wanted to clobber one.

A friend called Ron one evening and asked if he could come over. We straightened his room and I fixed some snacks. Martin let the boy in and came to the kitchen. In a few minutes we heard the front door close. "Never mind fixing anything," Ron called. "He's gone."

"He just got here," Martin said. "Why did he leave so soon?"

Ron stood in the doorway, leaning on his crutches. "He didn't have time to visit. It seems he lost his military whistle and wanted to borrow mine."

"Did you loan it to him?"

"Why not?" he said, shrugging in a sad, hopeless gesture. "I don't have much use for it." He turned to Kathy. "Hey, how about one of those crazy games you like to play. Bet I can beat you!"

Kathy only needed one hint for her games and ran to get them. Soon Ron's deep laughter and Kathy's little girl giggles filled the house.

"Listen to that," I whispered to Martin. "Oh how I love the sound of those two." He held me, and for a few minutes I let myself believe everything was normal.

If I thought the boy was rude, I was soon to learn adults can be too. We were waiting to see the doctor the next day when I noticed an elderly lady staring at Ron's foot. He had noticed her too.

"What did you do to that foot, young man?" she asked in a loud voice.

"I hurt it."

"Probably out kickin' a football when you should have been working. That's the trouble with young folks now days. They just . . ." She stopped when she saw the look on my face.

The nurse called Ron's name before I could say anything. When we were in the treatment room, Ron chuckled. "You know what I was about to tell her when the nurse called me? I was going to tell her I hurt my foot kicking a snoopy old lady."

He was laughing when the doctor came in. "I'm glad to see you in such a happy mood. That blood count is climbing back up there. Another massive dose should show more changes in those tumors." He sent Ron to the lab and asked me to wait in his office.

"I wanted to show you these X-rays of his lungs," he said. "This is the X-ray before we started the treatment. Here is the last one. See how much more noticeable they are in the first one."

"Then it's working!"

"For the present. But remember his body could start building up an immunity to the drugs. What we're doing is buying time. One extra week can mean a new drug. He's taken the treatment better than some adults do. That guy's a fighter."

As soon as the blood count was up, Ron returned to the hospital. They put him on the same floor and he was in a room with two men. One was elderly and very ill. I dreaded the second day, fearing depression would start.

When I went in, there was a big pot of flowers on his stand. "Look what the neighbors sent me," he said. "Wasn't that nice?" The drugs didn't cause depression as they had before.

One evening when Martin came from the hospital, I knew something was bothering him. "Is Ron worse?"

"No, it's me. I don't usually blow up at people. But I sure did tonight. The wife of the guy next to Ron walked out with me, harping all the way to the parking lot about how we were spoiling him. Her son was with her. Honey, I couldn't take any more. I said, 'Tell me something. If your son here had been given three months to live and the three months had passed, wouldn't you spoil him a little? I hope we have a long time left to love Ron and give him little things to make him happy.'

"She apologized and said they hadn't realized there was anything serious. He looked so healthy."

I held Martin close and let him cry it out. He's a person who holds his feelings inside too long. "Maybe that's been Ron's trouble," I said. "He was so healthy looking the doctors didn't think he was ill."

There was good news the next day. The tumor in his foot was smaller and a large one on his chest was almost gone. "Mom, I think they've got it whipped," Ron said, excitement and hope lighting his face. "My blood count hasn't dropped one bit. Isn't it the best news we've had?"

The progress continued into the fourth week. When I went in one afternoon he handed me a bill. "They said our insurance has run out. You're supposed to go talk to the business office. Mom, what are we going to do? Look how much it costs each day."

"You stop worrying. I'll go see what's wrong. The insurance isn't out yet."

My mind was in a daze. How could we have figured wrong? We were sure there was another five days left. Our insurance paid so many days or up to a certain amount. Since Ron's room was below the daily rate, the insurance would pay the set amount. But there was no way I could convince the business office of this. They insisted our insurance was out except for some medication.

"Look," I said, "you'll get your money. We'll pay what the insurance doesn't. Just don't take the bills to my son."

On Saturday, Martin visited Ron in the afternoon. He mentioned that the elderly man was worse. By the time I got there, he seemed better and his family went home.

Just before visiting hours were over, Ron mentioned the man's strange breathing. I went over and pulled the curtain back. He was choking. I ran into the hall. No nurse was in sight. An aide in another section went for help. It was several minutes before anyone came.

"If I get worse, will you stay with me?" Ron asked.

After what I had just seen there would be no doubt about it. We'll stay any time you ask." I hated to leave, but Ron assured me he was feeling OK.

Martin went the next afternoon and remarked that Ron was upset. The man had died and his family hadn't been notified until after his death. Once again, I regretted not listening to my conscience. I had debated about calling the daughter, but thought the hospital would.

When I got to Ron's room that evening, the other patient pointed to the bathroom. "He's in there. I think he's sick."

"Ron," I called through the door, "what's wrong?"

"The nurse said it was the malt Dad brought me. But it's a different kind of pain." He opened the door and I helped him into bed.

"Describe how you feel," I said. When he finished, I went to the nurse's station.

The nurse looked up. "Does your son need something?"

"Yes, I think he's having a reaction to one of the drugs he's getting."

"Oh," she said cooly, "are you a nurse?"

"No, but I have had a reaction from a drug he's taking. It was exactly like the pain Ron has."

"I can't give him any medication without the doctor's orders."

"I wouldn't want you to give him anything without calling Dr. Jordon first."

"This is Sunday. I'm not going to bother the doctor when I don't think it's necessary."

"You either call him or I will," I said, reaching for the phone.

"Oh, I'll do it!" She glared at me as she dialed. I heard Dr. Jordon answer and went back to Ron.

He reached up and grabbed my hand. "It hurts something awful, Mom. What's wrong with me?"

"Do you remember the time I had that bad reaction from a drug?" He nodded as the nurse came in with a shot.

"I'm sorry about this," she said. "I thought it was something else. The doctor really blasted me. I'll know better next time. But you know, some doctors get mad if you call them on Sunday no matter what happens. Dr. Jordon sure is different."

Within a few minutes the pain eased. "Mom, when I go home this time, I don't want to come back to the hospital. That poor old man died without his family last night. There should be some dignity in death."

I washed his head with a cool cloth. "You should rest now."

"Rest is all I do," he said sadly. "I want you to read a poem I wrote last night. Do you remember the piece in yesterday's paper about that teen-ager involved in a bad wreck? I knew him," he said, handing me the poem.

SHOW OFF

Take the car away from a show-off kid,
And you may save his life.
It's just the same in his immature hands
As a gun or a switch-blade knife.

Take his car away and he has nothing left—
He can't show off for his gang.
His teachers can tell you the type he is,
And he's really up on his slang.

Have you stopped lately to talk to your son,
Or do you have too much to do?
Do you really think you could talk very long?
Has he anything in common with you?

You'll look back soon and see your mistakes,
You gave in to every whim.
Was it when you gave him the car,
Or just didn't have time for him?

It's not the fault of the boy or the car—
They're not entirely to blame.
If you'd had the time to love him a lot
Do you think he'd turned out the same?

Are you proud of this kind of boy
As he runs through life rough-shod?
Do you ever wonder if he'd die today
Just how he would rate with God?

"It has a good message for parents," I said.

Ron was thoughtful for a few minutes, then said, "I really resented guys like him when I first got sick. But now, I don't know. Maybe I feel sorry for them. I'm not sure what they're trying to prove."

The blood count dropped rapidly each day and the medication had to stop. One morning Ron called to see why I hadn't picked him up. The hospital hadn't called me. Ron had his bag packed and was waiting in the hall when we got there. Kathy carried his bag and we went to the business office to settle the bill.

"Here's what you owe us," the clerk said.

"Can't we do as we've always done? You usually wait until the insurance comes back, then we pay the balance."

"Not when the bill is this high. Besides, your insurance has run out. If you can't pay, talk to the manager. He'll make arrangements."

Inside the manager's office, I explained that we had to draw money from savings. There wasn't enough in checking to cover the bill. He remained impersonal, insensitive to any suggestion that we wait until the insurance company settled or that I postdate the check. He seemed to enjoy his official, rubber-stamp duties and argued over an hour about this sudden change in their policy. I finally signed a note.

"You call this a religious affiliated hospital," I snapped, "and you can't trust me long enough to go to the bank."

"We should add another day," he said. "It's past check out time."

I stood up. "Don't push your luck. And don't sell that note to a loan company. My husband will pick it up."

During the drive home, Ron discovered we had been

charged for take-home drugs he didn't get. I knew what medication he was supposed to have, and we had been overcharged $15.

As soon as Ron was settled at home, I went to the bank. The loan department said our clear home would be collateral for loans we needed. I changed the savings to checking, wondering how long it would last. What would happen when our savings ran out? The two cars wouldn't bring as much as the past four weeks had cost. Would our house go next?

Middle income persons, unlike the rich or poor, have a disadvantage in obtaining sufficient health insurance. The family in the middle is ineligible for federal aid or free medical care. And they don't have the money to pay for the high medical costs. We had never dreamed how a long-term illness could break a family financially as well as emotionally.

Martin was home when I got back. "Give me the check book," he said. "I'm going to have a talk with Mr. Know-it-all at the hospital. I called the insurance company. They said over half of this bill was covered. He's also going to deduct the drugs we didn't get."

It was July. We had bought a few more months for Ron. But what a terrible price he had paid in suffering.

Chapter 9
Nuggets of Gold

Overlooked beauty and shunned opportunities can pass before our unseeing eyes when the mind is filled with pain or grief. But Ron missed very little.

He often surprised visitors, and usually greeted them with a cheerful remark and shared something he had read or seen. Little things that made up the interesting potpourri of his days brought laughter to some who came expecting to cry.

He continually searched his Bible for passages with messages for him. "You should try it sometime, Mom. It's like finding little nuggets of gold. Some information put there long ago jumps out with a special message just for you."

People were amazed that he never seemed bored. He loved to draw and write, often calling me to look at something. "Let me know if I'm a nuisance," he would say after calling me to his room. There was no way he could know how much we wanted to do for him. I would have gladly suffered the side effects the drugs had on him—the attacks of nausea, dizzy spells, and the loss of hair.

His healthy thick growth of hair grew thinner. He knew it was the medication and accepted it. One day he was in the bathroom a long time. I heard the thump thump of his crutches as he came to the kitchen. "Mr. Clean at your service, Ma'am," he said, grinning like a small boy.

I almost dropped the bowl in my hands as I stared at his bald head. "What did you do?" I gasped.

"Shaved my head. I don't like shedding. Don't you like the 'Mr. Clean' look?"

"I guess I'm stuck with it," I said, trying to be grateful he could still find humor in life. He was the family clown. No disease was going to make him lose that wonderful sense of humor.

We had grown accustomed to his bald head by the time we went back to the doctor. Even I had to laugh at the shocked look on people's faces when they saw him.

Dr. Jordon kept extensive records on each patient. When a patient went to the examination rooms, the records were placed in the room. The nurse rubbed Ron's head as she put his records on the table. "Take your shirt off, Yul Brynner. I'll be right back."

Instead of sitting down, Ron turned to the table. He pulled something from his pocket, spread it out on the charts, then cupped his hand over his mouth making choking sounds as the nurse walked in.

"Oh, no!" she gasped. "Not on the charts." That plastic mess again! The nurse started wiping the charts before she realized it was fake. "You stinker!" she scolded. "The only way I'll forgive you is for you to do it when I send the other nurse in."

Everyone loves a joke, and before the doctor got there Ron had played his trick on the entire staff.

Once again, Ron's blood count had reached the point where the medication started. "I don't want to go back to the hospital," he said. "Our insurance is out. Even if it wasn't, I would feel the same. Hospitals are depressing, noisy, and don't give the good service I get at home."

"I'll admit you do better at home. But what about your mother?" the doctor asked, looking at me. "Her back bothers her a lot. Can she take the strain?"

"I'd rather have him home," I said. "But if you think he'd be better off in the hospital, we'll get the money."

Dr. Jordon thought it over. "If you can bring him here once a week for the injections, I see no reason he can't stay home."

Ron was happier at home for many reasons. But the main one was his records. He loved all types of music, but two of his favorite singers were Jim Reeves and Marty Robbins. I heard their voices so much I almost thought of them as family. Ron would play their records and tape his voice in with them. I loved the tapes and encouraged him to make more.

"Not today," he said. "Marty, Jim and I are too tired. We've had a big recording session. You know, some day I'm going to write to them and tell them how much I've enjoyed their company these past months."

"Why don't you write now?"

"I'd only get a letter from a secretary. They'd be too busy to write."

He was listening to his radio the day they announced Jim Reeves' plane had crashed. Ron sat holding one of Jim's albums. "It doesn't seem fair," he said, putting the record on. When the record reached the song "Supper Time," Ron turned is face to the wall. I wasn't sure if he was crying or saying good-bye to a friend he'd never met.

The record ended and he turned it off. "Remember how I loved that song when I was little? I guess God decided it was time for Jim Reeves to come home. It'll be a lot nicer in Heaven with Jim there to sing."

Sadness over Jim Reeves' death stayed with him for several weeks. The cancer seemed to be in remission, but the injections continued. He had days when he was terribly nauseated and questioned the wisdom of taking any medicine. Then, the good days would come, giving him hope.

Fall was beautiful that year. Each time I had Ron out, I would drive him through areas where the trees were a riot of color. On an Indian summer day, we drove through the park, and he asked me to stop near some pines. "Remember how we used to gather pine cones for decorations?" he asked, with a sadness in his voice.

I nodded, remembering the good times. We were silent for a while, taking in the sheer beauty of nature. Geese flew over, headed south. "Look," Ron said, pointing to them. "Isn't it something the way they fly in formation?" His thoughts turned back to the trees. "I would like to have a nursery some day. It's a great feeling of accomplishment to grow things."

People had criticized us for letting Ron hope for a future. How can anyone say to someone they love, "You don't need to plan for tomorrow. You're going to die." I couldn't do it. In fact, we encouraged him to make plans for things he wanted to do. It kept his mind active. And then, we hoped he would get well. Scripture tells us: "Ask, and it shall be given you" (Matt. 7:7).

Thousands of people were asking God to spare Ron's life.

"Hey, how about taking me up to see the fellows in ROTC?" Ron asked, eager to see his friends.

I let him out near the door, hoping he wouldn't get caught in the hall during class change. He didn't stay long. As he reached the car, he turned and stood looking back at the school.

"Did you forget something?" I asked.

"No, a strange feeling came over me. Almost as though I had closed a door on that part of my life." He didn't talk much that evening. I'm sure he had to sort out his thoughts, trying to understand the feeling of finality he had at times.

When I went in to tell him good-night, he gave me this poem.

AFRAID

I had a friend when I was little,
I thought he was so brave;
He could whip a guy twice his size—
And I was his willing slave.
I won't use his real name here,
I'll just call him Joe.
All of us looked up to him,
There was nothing he didn't know.
Mom didn't approve of the things he did,
Nor some of the things he'd say.
She said everyone was afraid of something
And Joe would be some day.

As we grew older and started high school
Our paths didn't seem to cross.
I guess I'd grown sort of independent,
And Joe just had to be boss.

Then I got sick and left school,
And Joe was expelled for a fight.
I couldn't understand him any more;
He always knew he was right.
I hoped he'd stop when he drove by
But he never seemed to have time.
It's hard to remember that a few years ago
He was a good friend of mine.

I met him today when I went to school—
He didn't look me in the eye.
I knew now why he wouldn't come:
Someone told him I was going to die.
He just waved his hand and hurried on,
And I had quite a surprise.
I couldn't believe what I had seen—
I saw fear in Joe's eyes.
This tough guy had done some things
That made me catch my breath;
I knew now that he had a fear—
Joe was afraid of death.

This fellow I'd thought so brave
Was really a coward at heart.
I'd come to know God and to seek what
    was right—
This was why we'd grown apart.
I hadn't approved of Joe's wild ways,
And I'm glad of the choice I made.
God gave me the courage I need now
And without Him, Joe is afraid.

"What happened today at school?" I asked.

Ron shrugged, trying to control himself. "It was like I said in the poem. Most of the guys acted fine. But some, well, I get sick of people burying me. I'm not dead! I don't have a contagious disease. But a few sure act like it. And another thing, these well meaning Christians who are so worried about my soul had better worry about their own." His voice caught in a sob, and the mood stayed with him several days.

Things picked up for Ron the next week when his sergeant brought him his first lieutenant promotion. It was a wonderful gesture from them and Ron was proud.

We had planned the usual family Thanksgiving. By the time I had dinner on, Ron was too ill to eat anything. Everyone was eating, while I was dying a little inside. It didn't seem right with Ron so sick. There was no way I could tell the guests to go home.

Within two days, edema was so bad he had to borrow some of Martin's clothes to wear to the doctor. More medicine. When the edema left, I could tell he had lost a lot of weight.

Ron had started writing in a journal. "I want you to read this some day," he said. "It's just thoughts I've put down. Did you know writing is a good way to relieve anguished minds?"

"Do you have an anguished mind?"

"Yes, sometimes in the middle of the night. You know, when the train goes through the valley wailing that lonesome sound, my mind feels the same way—like a lost soul crying out in anguish. Does that make any sense to you, Mom?"

"Yes, I've felt the same way."

"Sometimes I feel so rotten, I wonder if I'll ever get better. But then I remember how much pain I had before they started the shots. I want to live. But there was a time I thought of committing suicide. I know that's wrong. Have you ever had such thoughts?"

I told him about the time I stood at the river, asking

God to give me one reason. "You were the reason, Son. God meant for you to be born. He had a purpose for you."

A smile played across his lips. "That gives me a good feeling to think I saved your life. As for my purpose, I've been thinking about that—trying to find out my reason for being." He started coughing. Once the coughing stopped, he continued, "Between my hacking and Taffy's moaning, I'll bet Dad doesn't get much sleep. You'd better take her to a vet. She sounds awful sick."

Taffy was 13 years old, blind and had moaned continuously during the past week. Even with all of our bills, there was nothing left to do but take the last sad trip for what I knew would be the veterinarian's lethal shot. Taffy licked my hand as though she knew it was goodbye. How I dreaded telling Ron and Kathy.

"What did the vet say?" Ron called when he heard me come in. I didn't need to answer. He knew when he saw me. "Don't cry," he said, pulling my head down on his shoulder. "She's had a good life—and a long one. I knew she was in awful pain."

Kathy had been sure Taffy would get better. Her dog's death was a shock. But knowing what her brother was going through made the grief pass. That night she thanked God for the years we'd had Taffy.

I knew Kathy prayed often for Ron as we all did. But I don't think anyone talked to God as much as Ron. His prayer and meditation made him seem far older. He showed a deep faith that we hadn't realized existed in our happy-go-lucky son. Beneath his humorous exterior was a very deep person.

One day a group of teen-age boys were going by our house. They were yelling and hitting one another. I couldn't help thinking, *why my son?*

Ron must have seen the look on my face. He gently reached up and patted my arm. "Mom, don't be bitter about this. You wouldn't wish them any harm. There comes a time in each person's life when science can't help. Maybe that's what has happened this time.

"Be grateful for what we've had. You know the four of us have something rather special. Whatever the future holds, nothing can take that away. I . . ." He started coughing and I ran for his medicine.

The coughing subsided and he lay his head back in the chair and closed his eyes. He looked so tired. "I know the coughing is from the tumors in my lungs. They don't have to tell me those things. It's strange, how you sense things that aren't said."

Kathy came in just then and his mood changed. He seemed determined not to let her see him during the bad times. That was why she didn't actually realize how ill he was.

Tears started forming and I clamped my eyes tight to stop them. After all those months, one would think there wouldn't be any tears left. But there always seemed to be a few more to surface at the wrong time.

"Do you feel like giving me my spelling words?" Kathy asked him.

"Sure," Ron said. "But let me warn you, I'll be worse than any teacher. Just hesitate on one letter and I'll count it wrong."

I hurried to the hitchen on the pretense of checking dinner. The kitchen and laundry room had become my places for quiet prayer.

Former neighbors came to visit Ron that evening. Their daughter, Jeanie, had changed from a thin, quiet child into a beautiful teen-ager—and Ron noticed.

Jeanie had a bubbly personality and they were soon

off to themselves catching up on the years since they had played together. They stayed late, and Ron didn't want the evening to end.

"I'll come again," Jeanie promised. "During the holidays I'll spend an afternoon with you."

Ron talked about Jeanie for days. "I wish I had called her to attend some of the things at school. She sure is an interesting person."

"She's also pretty," I said.

"Yeah, I noticed," he answered, an impish grin spreading across his face.

Christmas was approaching, and I tried to force myself to get in the spirit of a season we had found so joyous. Martin was working two and sometimes three jobs to meet expenses. I had tried working a night shift in a factory during the summer. After two nights, I realized Ron wasn't asking for help during the day to let me sleep.

Ron still talked about starting a nursery when his foot got better. Maybe it was dreams, but that hope for a future kept him going. One of Martin's jobs was at an experimental laboratory, and he brought Ron some little trees they had dumped. One was a tiny fir and the others were mugho pines. The pines looked sick so Martin planted them. Ron put the fir by his bed. "I've named him Sam," he said. "That stands for save America's mughos."

"Sam isn't a mugho pine; I think it's a fir."

"It doesn't matter. Sam is a good name. He'll be the most beautiful tree in my nursery. I'll plant him at the entrance."

Sam's limbs started drooping that week. "Mom, plant him in the garden where he'll be protected this winter," he instructed. After Sam was planted, we got a small

Christmas tree for Ron's room. He made a tiny blinking star from things in his closet.

We made a trip to the doctor that week that made me have nightmares. Ron's veins would not take the needles. After 23 times they gave up. I'd had to leave the room because I was ill. My tears matched the rain, as I stood looking out the window. *Why does it always have to rain when we come here,* I thought. *Does the world cry with us?*

The doctor came out. "I can't do this to him. We'll have to switch to oral medicine. It isn't as effective, but this isn't fair to him."

"The tumors are getting worse, aren't they?"

"Yes, but it did slow them down for several months."

"Ron thinks the tumors in his lungs are getting larger."

"They probably are. I want to take an X-ray. He won't need to come back until after New Years."

Ron came out and leaned against the wall. "Doc, do you make house calls?"

"Yes, why?"

"I may get to a point where I can't make it in."

Dr. Jordon put his arm around Ron's shoulders as they went to X-ray. "I'll come any time you need me."

The rain had stopped when we left, and a rainbow looked as though it had gift wrapped the world. "Look!" Ron exclaimed. "Do you remember how God put the rainbow in the sky as a sign to Noah? Maybe this rainbow is a sign for us. You'll have to admit they are unusual this time of the year."

How could a rainbow offer me hope? I had seen the look on the nurse's face when Ron said he might not be able to come in. *Oh, God,* my mind screamed, *I feel like giving the wheel a quick turn and ending it all. Why didn't you let me jump in the river that day? What was the reason for his life? He has to gasp for every breath, suffer agonizing pain–and for what reason? God–are You even listening?*

"You know," Ron said, breaking into my depressing thoughts, "People have to look for the rainbows in life. The little bits of happiness that happen to us each day—they're the rainbows God sends us. We just have to watch for them."

I thought about that for a few minutes, then replied, "Young man, you are beautiful."

"You only say that because my hair has grown out. You never said bald is beautiful."

He asked me to stop on the way home and buy his Christmas present for Kathy. "Get her something with a mustard seed," he said. "They had them advertised."

I picked out a necklace with one mustard seed suspended in a plastic ball. "Is this what you had in mind?" I asked, handing him the package and his change.

He examined the necklace. It looked tiny in his hand. "Yes, this will do. The Lord said, 'If you have faith as a grain of mustard seed . . .' Kathy will understand."

The trip sapped his strength completely that day. Was there something he wasn't telling me? I wondered how much pain we never knew about.

Christmas had been a time we had enjoyed giving to others. But there wouldn't be groceries or toys for a needy family. For the first time we had to be on the receiving end. People sent money and gifts to Ron. Friends and strangers sent him money to buy what he wanted. One group of young people bought him a record album. Another group fixed a big box with a gift for each day of the next month. But like a little kid, Ron had Kathy pull each gift out until all of them were opened.

Maybe it was the spirit of Christmas helping him or perhaps he was pretending for Kathy's sake, but it was meaningful. We watched the two of them working intently on a puzzle. Martin reached for my hand. My mind said over and over, *please, Lord, let it last.*

I tried to remember some Scripture that might help. Like Ron, the Psalms helped me, too. "Cast thy burden upon the Lord, and He shall sustain thee" (Psalm 55:22).

Ron was right. They were like finding little nuggets of gold on the barren desert of life.

Chapter 10
For Everything There Is a Season

Bright sunlight played hopscotch across Ron's bed when I went in to wish him happy birthday.

"What kind of cake do you want?" I asked, planting a kiss on his cheek.

He gave me a hug that started a bad coughing spell. When it ended he lay exhausted. "Would you mind just staying in my room and talking? I'd rather you and Kathy talk to me than bake a cake I can't eat. I feel more like 100 than 17 today."

"What do you want to talk about?"

"All the good times we've had." And Ron began to search his memory for treasures we had long forgotten. "Remember . . ." There was the time he had complained because so many friends were out of town on his birthday. I had promised to let him have a party later. Finally, a special day arrived. School was going to let out at noon. Since he was eight, that would be a good number to invite. But Ron didn't know who could come so he announced it during class. I ended up with all of them. "That party was a big surprise on you, Mom."

Kathy soon joined our day of good memories. I fixed us a lunch we could eat in Ron's room. He ate very little, but he was enjoying his day.

Good days, like Christmas and his birthday, seemed to give him a spiritual lift, releasing him from his painful body. But it ended the next day when he started passing blood and having severe pains in the bladder. Another type of medicine—another kind of pain.

Dr. Jordon warned us that any infection could take Ron in a few hours. Jeanie had the flu over the holidays, making it impossible for her to visit.

On New Year's Eve I went to his room to ask Ron if he could eat. Martin was fixing hamburgers. Ron was listening to the radio and shushed me until he heard the weather report. "Now," he said, reaching over to turn off the radio, "I'll take a nice . . . a nice . . ." His head drew back and his body started jerking and twisting.

"Help me!" I screamed.

Martin and Kathy ran into the room. Martin tried to hold Ron on the bed. "Call the doctor quick!"

My fingers were shaking so hard I could barely dial the phone. "Dr. Jordon," I cried, "something is wrong with Ron. He can't control his body."

I heard Martin cry out, "I think he's dead." Kathy started crying. I hung up and ran to Ron. We listened for a heartbeat. "He's alive!" Martin cried. "I hope the doctor gets here in case it starts again."

It was only a short time before Dr. Jordon came. He examined Ron and gave him a shot. We waited. Ron finally opened his eyes. "What are you doing here, Doc?"

"Thought I'd drop in and help you celebrate New Year's Eve."

"What happened? The last thing I remember was talking to Mom. What made me pass out?"

"You're probably not getting enough oxygen. I'll order some out tonight."

Dr. Jordon turned to me. "Will you show me where the telephone is?" He ordered the oxygen and motioned me to the kitchen.

"What happened?" I asked, my teeth chattering.

"I told him the truth. His brain isn't getting enough oxygen. What he had was a grand mal seizure. There could be a tumor in his brain. When we X-rayed his lungs last time, I could understand the bad cough. Frankly, I don't know how he's breathing. His lungs are full of tumors. Most likely, it's tumors in his bladder."

"Are you giving up?"

"No," he said, wiping his eyes, "as long as we have him, there's hope. But you've got to get control of yourself. He needs you."

"Will he have to go back to the hospital? Our insurance is in effect, but I'd rather keep him at home."

The doctor shook his head. "He's happier here. I promised him he could stay home as long as you can care for him. The lack of privacy, the loneliness, and the thought I'd gone back on my promise to him would only serve to dehumanize him a little more.

"Here in his home he has a connection with his past life, an active present life when he feels like it, and God willing, a future."

At that time it was costing far more to keep Ron home than in the hospital. Our insurance would have paid for the oxygen and medication in a hospital but not at home. Many thought our decision stupid. Right or wrong, we had to let Ron make the choice. Had he realized the difference in cost, I'm sure he would have gone to the hospital. But I had to make sure we did what he wanted. I said it wouldn't be much cheaper in the hospital. Home was his choice.

Although Ron could operate the oxygen when he needed it, he wasn't to be left alone for long. I started sleeping where I could see his bed. He didn't sleep much and usually read or wrote in his journal.

One night I was reading in his room after Martin and Kathy had gone to bed. "I've got a poem for Dad's birthday. Do you want to read it?"

TO A NICE GUY

You were always such a nice guy—
To me you seemed so smart.
At times I tried your patience
And almost broke your heart.

I would rassle you and love you
And ride upon your back.
I knew when I got out of line
I'd get a good sound smack.

You taught me so many things
And helped me through the years.
Sometimes you were so proud
Your eyes would fill with tears.

My one goal in all these years
Was not to be a better man.
But just to make you proud of me—
With God's help, I'm sure I can.

Thanks doesn't seem sufficient
For all the things you've done.
Dad, I'm sure you'll always know
That I'm proud to be your son.

"That's beautiful," I said, wiping away my tears.

"It's the way I feel. We did a good job in picking him. Mom, no matter how bad I get, promise you won't call that other guy . . . What's his name?"

"Bob. I wouldn't call him. In the first place, I wouldn't have any idea where he is."

Ron didn't say anything for a long time. I knew from the way he was acting something was bothering him. "There's something I should have told you years ago. I knew you'd be mad at me.

"One time in the third grade I was taking papers to school. I dropped them and a man stopped and asked if he could take them to school for me. I thought he was one of the guys working on the new houses in back of us. After I got in the car, I recognized him from the picture you had shown me. He asked me all sorts of questions. Did I like my dad? Was he good to me? Did I mind my mother?

"It was strange looking at a man I should have had some feeling for. But there was nothing. If I felt anything it was pity. How lonesome he must be.

"When we got to school, I slid out the door. 'Thanks, Mister,' I said, and hurried up the steps. He probably thought I was thanking him for the ride. But what I was really saying was 'Thanks, for staying out of our lives.' Confession time is over," Ron said, looking relieved. "Now you can spank me."

"There was too much of that, I'm afraid. Son, I'm sorry I was so strict on you. I didn't want you to grow into a person like Bob."

Ron reached out and took my hands. "Let's face it, Mom, I was a stinker. When I see the way some of the kids turned out, I'm glad you and Dad cared enough to make me mind. To some kids, discipline is a dirty word.

Without it, I couldn't have made it these past months."

He had to use the oxygen mask before he could finish. "Whatever happens with me, don't change toward Kathy. Teen-agers need someone to make them keep the rules."

He was so quiet, I thought he had gone to sleep. "I have another confession to make," he said. "There were times, when I first got sick, I questioned the existence of God. Some people say there is no God. I found myself wondering, what if they're right? What if there is nothing when we die? But now, I feel an inner voice tell me He's standing so close I say, 'Good morning, God.' When I meditate, this Source reveals things I never took time to think about before."

Ron was sorting out his thoughts, trying to help me understand. But he was on a higher state of consciousness, touching levels I'd never dared dream of. Ron was tuned in to something I could not share. His spiritual sensitivity gave him the ability to see the unseen and hear with an inner ear that hears the whispering of the earth most of us miss.

At that moment, God gave me a glimpse into a very beautiful soul, and I was proud of what I saw.

The next afternoon Ron finally got some sleep. I heard him call out and hurried to his room as Kathy came in from school. "Mom, do you feel another presence in the room?" he asked.

I sensed something but wasn't sure what I felt.

Ron handed me a pencil and paper. "Will you write this down as I try to recall it? I'm not sure if it was a dream or . . . Anyway, a man was taking me and a blind girl along a path. I told him, 'Go slow. I can't walk on crutches.'

"He said, 'From here on, you can walk.'

"I could walk without crutches and the girl could see. We walked with a weightless feeling through misty clouds, traveling the distance in sort of a 'thought transport.' The man pointed to a door across a deep chasm and we were instantly there.

"Inside, people greeted me. Not in words but in thoughts. I knew some of them. A lady had me hang something on a wall and I fell. It didn't hurt and the people told me I'd soon get used to the difference.

"I told the people I wanted to leave. The girl I'd come with said she didn't want to go back to being blind. The people told me, 'Don't you understand? You can't go back.'

"Everyone knew my thoughts and gave me directions. I ran up a long narrow stairway to a large room. A lot of people sat at a long table. The man who had brought me there came forward.

"He took my hands and welcomed me. I told him, 'I can't stay here. I have too many things to do. My family will be looking for me.'

"The man smiled. 'Return for now. But when we call again, you must come.'

"There was a rushing of air and I felt like my body was transported through a tunnel. I opened my eyes and felt something in my room. Sheba must have felt it because she looked wild-eyed and ran out like she was scared. But Sol got up in my arms like he is now."

Sol was curled in Ron's lap. One little paw gently reached up, touching Ron on the cheek. Their eyes met in an emotional outpouring of love.

There was something in Ron's room—something special. Kathy felt it, too. I felt the splendor of real spiritual awareness beyond anything I'd felt before—beyond any dimension I'd ever touched. Part of me felt as Sheba must have felt—a little scared of the unseen. But another part of me, a part I often ignored, felt the emotion Sol was showing. I could see a glow of light around both of them, or thought I did. It must be imagination.

A warm feeling came over me. I wanted to hold time still, but the telephone broke the spell. Kathy answered it for me.

"Mom, do you think I saw Jesus?" Ron asked. "I can't remember what the man looked like."

"I think you've been very close to Jesus for a long time, Ron." Was this God's way of showing him he had nothing to fear?

He sat quiet for a few minutes. "You may as well go talk to whoever's on the phone. If you don't, they'll think I'm worse and call half the town. Sometimes I wish we didn't have a telephone."

Unfortunately, he was right. But we had to have the phone to call the doctor. During Ron's illness, I almost hated the sound of a telephone. At least the calls offering false hopes had stopped. Someone would hear of a doctor who had cured cancer and call me before checking it out. My hopes would zoom high. After they found it wasn't true, my hopes would drop to zero, and I'd die a little inside. But that call was beyond belief.

"Mrs. Butler," the crisp voice said. "This is the administrator of the hospital your son was in. I understand you were angry about us making you pay the bill."

I explained what had happened. "That was six months ago," I said. "What difference does it make now?"

"You had no business telling others about this! Because of you, one church cut off their donation to us. Your insurance company was also angry."

"The church that cut you off was a relative's church. They didn't do it because of us. It happens that several of the members had been treated the same way. Don't you think people have a right to some dignity when they are trying to pay their bills? As for the insurance company, I don't blame them. Your staff had no business making us pay before the insurance company settled."

"I'm telling you right now," she shouted, "you'd better not cause another church to withdraw funds."

By then I was crying. "Please," I whispered, "I had nothing to do with that church. Do you have any idea what we're going through? Don't you know what's wrong with our son?"

"I don't care what's wrong with him. That's not my job. If you have another complaint, you come to me."

"Don't worry, I will. And believe me, it will be an experience you won't forget," I said, hanging up on her.

Ron had turned his radio on, so he hadn't heard the conversation. Kathy hugged me, trying to calm me. She was crying, too, sure it had been more bad news about Ron. I was finally able to explain. "Go to your room and cry," she said. "I'll stay out here in case Ron needs something."

"Oh, God," I sobbed into my pillow, "please keep me from hating people like her." After my crying was over, Kathy placed a wet cloth over my eyes.

"Try to sleep," she said. "I told Ron you were going to rest. He's reading, so I'll do some of the ironing for you." She held me close, comforting me as I had done so many times when she was hurting.

Ron talked more about his dream that night. "Do you think there is communication between God and us . . . like maybe through dreams . . . at least for directions?"

"Yes," I said, reminding him of Dad's warning about the steps.

"I've been reading about people who have experienced it. You know, a mother and her children are of the same body. I think that would be the closest link between the two worlds. Take us, we're a lot alike in our thinking. Don't you think if one of us would die there would be a good possibility of communication through Jesus . . . for comfort?"

Before I could answer, Martin came in from work. "Go fix something warm for Dad to eat," Ron said. "I know he's hungry."

It was after midnight and Martin had been working in the cold since morning. My heart ached for him. I wasn't sure which was worse—working long hours to pay the bills or watching Ron suffer. It worried me that Martin might collapse physically. Besides his long hours, he had to wrestle the heavy oxygen tanks up on the front porch. Not one man on the block offered to help him, and he wasn't the type to ask. With my arthritis growing worse each day, he wouldn't let me help.

After Martin ate, I went in to check Ron. He was thumbing through a book for a passage he'd read about death written by Norman Vincent Peale.

Martin came in to tell Ron good night. "I wish you had a better job, Dad. One where you didn't have to be out in the bad weather."

"It's not so bad," he assured him. Martin sat beside Ron for a while. "I'd better get some sleep, Son."

Ron was busy flipping pages. "There was something I wanted to show you. If I find it, I'll save it."

"I'll be here in the morning," Martin said.

"But I may not be," Ron answered.

Martin's eyes met mine. That was the first time Ron had made such a remark in front of his dad. I'm not sure Ron was aware of what he said. In his own way, he was trying to prepare us for something our minds wouldn't accept.

"Jeanie's mother called about you," I told him the next morning. "She said Jeanie came by last week, but a neighbor said you couldn't have visitors yet. Do you want me to have her come over?"

"No, I don't think so. I have my reasons." He placed the oxygen mask over his face and stared at the ceiling, lost in thought.

Later, he said, "It would be easy to love a girl like Jeanie. Why should I mess up her life? For a brief time, she brought something special to me. But right now, I can't see hurting us both."

Another snow storm had started. Ron pulled the curtains back so he could see the wind whipping the trees. "Did you put leaves around Sam? A storm like this could blow him away."

"The garage will protect him. It's you we need to keep warm," I said, pulling blankets over his legs.

He grinned up at me. "You worry like a mother hen. But you know something? I like it." Once again his thoughts went back to his tree. "Sam may not make it to spring," he said. "There will always be times we have to let go of people or things we love. It's hard for you to let go, isn't it, Mom?"

"Yes, it always has been. I try not to be that way. Maybe it's insecurity that makes me hold on. Then again, I could be selfish."

He gently patted my arm. "You're not selfish. I can vouch for that. It's only human to want to hold on to a special time or people—even pets."

"It was hard for me to give up Pal. He was so special to me. I was glad you didn't get another collie. That would have seemed as though you were trying to replace him. Taffy was a dignified little lady. The next dog should be an ornery type. They're a lot of company."

"Would you like a dog?"

"I wasn't thinking of one for myself. I was thinking of one for you—to keep you company."

A chill of apprehension washed over me. Was he preparing me for the tomorrows when he couldn't comfort me? *Oh, God, he loves life, and never wastes a minute. He lives each one to the fullest, with no time squandered on self-pity.*

Ron made a rough sketch of the dog he thought I needed. We both laughed. "He looks more like a little old man," Ron said, wadding up the drawing.

"I wish you wouldn't throw your sketches away."

He changed the subject. "What kind of day dreams did you have when you were young?"

"Like all kids, I was going to be rich."

"Did any of your dreams come true?"

"Of course. To me, being rich was having a new store-bought dress and all the fruit I wanted. And I always said I was going to have a good husband, a boy and a girl. That's the way it was in all the stories. Each family consisted of one boy and one girl. My parents goofed."

He laughed. "Your dreams were limited." Then he told me his dreams, places he went through "mind travel." "But that's enough about me, tell me more about the old days."

"I'll ignore that! In many movies, people went to the Waldorf Astoria in New York. Imagine a kid who had to scrounge all week to pay for a movie dreaming of staying at the Waldorf."

"I think you'll stay there some day," he said, pulling the drapes back. "Look at it snow. We don't want to go to New York tonight. Let's go to Hawaii. Man, I can just see those warm beaches. Imagine what it must be like underwater there." For a time, I think he walked the sandy beaches and explored the beauty of a world he would never see. Then he came back to me.

"I'd like to see both places. But why limit our 'mind travel.' Now we can dream about going to the moon."

"That will be the day! I don't think man is that smart. Besides, they can't handle this planet."

"Want to bet?" he asked, eager to get me into a discussion of a subject I had little knowledge of or faith in at that moment. "I'll bet they land on the moon and find a cure for cancer before 1970. Mom, you don't have enough faith in science."

He was right. It was rather a hard thing to believe in as I watched our son slowly slip away from us.

The coughing grew worse each day, he needed oxygen most of the time, and once more convulsions racked his body. I didn't see how he held out against the insidious disease which was mercilessly attacking each organ. One day he started to reach for a pen. I heard a snap as he groaned and held his ribs. "Mom, I think I broke something! It hurts!"

I called the doctor and told him what happened.

"The tumors are growing between the ribs. I'll have the druggist send you some elastic bandage to bind him. We'll have to increase the pain pills. Tell him I'll come by tomorrow."

When I returned to Ron, he was holding a blanket tight around him. Tears were misting his eyes. "It's tumors cracking my ribs, isn't it?" I nodded, not trusting myself to speak.

Wrapping him helped a little. The increase in drugs worried Ron. He was afraid of becoming addicted to them. This memory was going to make me bitter in later years.

There was little sleep for him. He couldn't lie down. Sleeping pills only gave him a few minutes rest. I slept in a chair in his room. Sometimes I read to him. His records and books were stacked neatly on a table as though he was through with them.

One night after we had finished the 23rd Psalm, he remarked, "I wonder if they would allow an ROTC cadet to be buried in his uniform if it was paid for? There's enough money left in my savings. Will you ask the sergeant?"

"Yes, if you want me to."

"I'd like for you to call the minister that baptized me. Do you know where he is?"

"I'm sure we have his address." That seemed to satisfy him. The next morning I mailed the letters telling them Ron was worse.

When the sergeant called, I told him what Ron had asked about the uniform. "Isn't there any hope?" he asked.

"I don't see how there can be," I whispered. "Hope has kept us going, but he can't take much more."

"Would you allow us to have a military funeral for him?"

"I . . . yes, that's the way he would want it."

"I'll come visit him tomorrow."

We just can't give up, I thought. *Miracles do come. Why not here, Lord, why not here?*

I took the paper to Ron. "I can't read it, Mom. I'm going blind."

"Maybe it's the medicine," I said, my heart sinking.

When Martin came in that evening, he said he wasn't going to work the next week. "I know we need the money, but I want some time with him." I told him about Ron's eyes, and we cried together.

Both the sergeant and our former pastor came the next

day. Ron reached over and shook hands with each one. The pastor prayed. Ron was in so much pain they didn't stay long.

Many people from all parts of the city were praying for Ron. Someone sent men from a denomination that uses the laying on of hands. "Do you mind if we have a prayer service for you?" they asked. Ron was unable to speak because of the oxygen mask. He held out his hands to the men. I had wanted to take him to another country for this. Had God decided to send us that miracle? Ron's breathing eased, he seemed at peace with the world, and he was able to thank the men for coming.

I had forgotten it was my birthday. Ron had a little gift Mom had bought for him to give me. "I wanted to get you something. They say life begins at 40. I'm sure not giving you a happy birthday."

My life wasn't beginning at 40. Part of it was slipping away before my eyes. *Oh, God,* my mind screamed, *it isn't fair! What was the purpose of his life if You take him now?*

Kathy asked us to leave them alone that evening. We could hear her crying and trying to tell Ron how much she loved him. They talked for a long time, then she kissed him and ran to her room.

"Doesn't Kathy realize how much I love her?" he asked when I went in. "I hope all of you realize how much you mean to me."

"We do, Ron. She thinks you are the greatest brother a girl ever had."

Sol had been curled in Ron's arms for hours. He slept there or curled at the foot of the bed except when I made him go out. I had wondered if it was all devotion or snacks from Ron's tray. But I knew as Ron grew worse. Sheba would only come to Ron's door. Sol glared at every person who came as if he thought they might take his friend away. I think he sensed death and like a little guard, he was trying to keep an unseen enemy away.

"Aren't you tired of holding him?" I asked.

Ron lovingly stroked Sol. "No, I don't get tired of holding him. Mom, promise you'll always take good care of him. No one else would understand him."

I promised and we sat in the darkened room. Sol's purr and the sound from the oxygen lulled me into a brief sleep. I was running wildly through a valley searching for a child. Those rasping sounds told me I had lived this dream before. My eyes flew open. The sound was Ron breathing. Had I dreamed of his death the day he was born?

Ron was looking at me. "It's strange, but lately when I do my mind travel I seem to always go to this beautiful bay. It's great for scuba diving." He described the place so vividly I felt as though he took me there.

During the night he drifted in and out of a coma. He asked Martin and I to lower him into the water. We didn't understand. "See it? . . . water is so blue . . . Help me down . . . so I can swim."

We held him as though lifting him into water. "Here we go, Son," Martin said.

Ron's eyes were closed, a contented smile came over his face as he made weak swimming motions. "It's beautiful here . . . Don't worry . . . I want to swim . . . across it."

By morning the pain was worse. Ron looked up at Martin and said, "Dad, it hurts so bad. Help me, please."

Martin called the doctor to see if he could give Ron a stronger drug. "He's in a coma," Dr. Jordon said.

Martin was crying. "Not all the time. He's rational enough to know us."

The new medicine helped, but Ron was partly conscious, still fighting to live, still holding on to life with what little strength he had. Why? Was he asking us to let him go when he wanted to swim? Was he asking our permission to leave? *I'll let go, God. Please, don't let him suffer any longer.*

When we gave Ron his medicine that afternoon, he said, "I know . . . it's almost time." Martin and I looked at each other across the thin boy who was taking part of us with him. It seemed as though he had felt my release and was ready to start a new journey.

The beautiful miracle we had known as our son slipped away that evening. His labored breathing stopped. Jesus reached out His hand and called, "Come home, Ron."

I took the limp hand I was holding, kissed the palm and gently closed his fingers around it as he had once done to me. "Hold on to that," I whispered, "and remember I love you."

Death used to be a private thing. Not any more. Ron had to be turned over to strangers. Be careful, I wanted to tell those white-coated men who carried our son away, that is someone special.

During the night I went to Ron's empty room and sat in the darkness trying to sort out my feelings. There was relief that his pain was over and anger that his life was cut short.

What if I'd agreed to an abortion or ended our lives in the river? What if I'd never known the 17 years of love, laughter and tears Ron brought into my life? Those years were worth the pain I felt. My "what if" was answered, but the guilt and anger stayed.

For everything there is a season . . . A time to live . . . A time to die . . . Part of me had died.

Chapter 11
Grief

It took several minutes for me to realize it was morning and to shake off the effects of sleeping pills. Rays of sun reached in around the shades, telling me it was our first day without Ron.

Shock comes with the death of a loved one, regardless of the length of illness. It numbed me, blocking out reality, as I went through the day in a zombie-like state. People came, asked questions. I answered. But inside, I was screaming, protesting.

Regardless of inward turmoil, we had to make plans. The sergeant met us at the funeral home. Ron would have a full military funeral. The paper printed his photograph and ROTC record with his death notice.

There will always be crackpots who dote on other people's troubles—who are against everything. At the time, I wasn't aware that families of men killed in Vietnam were being harrassed. Ours came in the form of unsigned letters that didn't make sense. Somehow, the fact Ron was in any way connected to the military must have made some think this was his punishment. But those few didn't bother us too much when we had so many letters from people who cared.

The best consolation we received was from people who had lost a child with cancer. Each letter started out the same: You don't know us, but our hearts and prayers are with you . . . They understood.

The funeral home visitation was something I dreaded. In a way, it helped. Ron's friends came to say "goodbye." There isn't time for this during a funeral, and we most likely would never have heard the little stories his friends told us about our son. One cadet told us how Ron had talked him into taking ROTC when he was thinking about dropping out of school. "Ron sure was some kind of a salesman," he said. "I'm glad I listened to him." Several cadets had moved and made a long trip back.

On the day of the funeral, we went out early to be alone. As we went into the funeral home, one of his teachers was leaving. "I didn't know until they announced his death at school," she said. "Students move away and I assumed Ron had. I wish I'd known. He was one of the sweetest students I've had. Ron had a special charisma—a charm about him—I see in some students. He would have gone far. It makes a person wonder why."

During the service, I tried not to look at the rows of ROTC cadets blinking back tears. Ron hadn't wanted them to know how ill he was. His senior year hadn't been the fun year he had looked forward to. It had been pain from his disease and disappointment that he had to forfeit his position as color guard commander.

Our former pastor started speaking. A tightness in my chest made me sick as Martin and Kathy grasped my hands. "This family was very close, always together. Now Ron has left them . . ." He hesitated, his voice breaking, then continued. "I woke up this morning, sad about coming here. But something happened that changed my mood.

"Ron was a fan of the late Jim Reeves, as many of us are. He was very upset when Jim was killed last year. Later, he remarked to his mother that Heaven would be even better with Jim Reeves there to sing. I turned on the radio as I headed toward the city. Jim Reeves was singing, 'Supper Time,' one of Ron's favorites. It reminded me that Heaven will be even better because Ron is there."

The funeral was over and we came to that last few moments as a family. Out of habit, I gently pushed Ron's hair back. *Oh, God,* I thought, *this is the last time I can touch that beautiful hair. His face doesn't look right without an impish grin.*

At the grave his friends conducted the military funeral. Ron had trained the cadet holding the American flag. Suddenly, a wind whipped the flag and almost blew it from the cadet's hands. Then, as abruptly as it had started, the wind died. Another cadet remarked, "I knew Ron wouldn't give up that flag without a fight."

The last sounds of the bugle echoed through the valley, and they presented me the flag that had draped his casket. My eyes clouded with tears, the colors blurred, giving it the appearance of a rainbow. I remembered Ron saying, "We have to look for our rainbows, Mom."

Was he right? Were there rainbows even in sadness? The night he died, the weather had been stormy. "Oh,

God," I had cried, "You know the horror I have of a funeral in bad weather." And the weather had changed, turning warmer.

People crowded around us offering sympathy. Some didn't know what to say, so they kept quiet. For them, we were grateful. Others didn't know what to say, so they uttered stupid, empty phrases like, "God knows best" or "It's God's will."

Each time someone mouthed those hollow words, I wanted to scream, "How would you know? You still have all of your children."

We went home, and friends and family came too. Kathy went to Ron's room, and I followed her. "They're in the kitchen eating and visiting as though this was a party," she cried, her voice rising hysterically. "Don't they know my brother is dead?"

"Honey, some of them have a long drive. With all the food people sent, wouldn't it be rather selfish not to share it?"

But there was no reasoning with her. She had felt Ron would make it. Right then, she was angry at everyone.

"I'll play his tapes," she sobbed. "At least we can hear his voice." The tape turned, but there wasn't any sound.

"Kathy," I said, gently pulling her away from the recorder, "there are no tapes with Ron's voice. I was going to play them last night. They're blank!"

"No! he had three tapes of him singing with his records," she cried.

"He must have erased them. There were empty tapes, so he must have planned on making these over—and time ran out."

It took her hours to play every tape, hoping his voice was on some. I heard her cry, "Oh, Ronnie, why did you do it? I wanted to at least hear you." Finally, hope gone and drained of tears, she put the tape player away.

Kathy seemed to adjust when she went back to school. Martin went back to work, and I had an empty house to hear me cry.

I sat in Ron's room for hours with the cats. They had been put downstairs a few hours before Ron's death and left there until after the funeral. Both cats seemed to connect the flag on Ron's bed to his disappearance. Sheba acted afraid of it, but we had found Sol clawing at the plastic flag cover and whimpering. He would also claw at Ron's pillow and make a meowing noise that sounded like a tiny baby crying. He searched the house, sure Ron was playing games with him.

The numb feeling that took me through Ron's illness, his death then the funeral, left. And in its place came the deep sense of loss.

The physical body of a loved one can no longer be seen, but something, call it spirit, soul or whatever, is still there. It fills every room, lingering on furniture or special articles—calling to the living in silence so loud it touches those who listen: *Hold me, love me, acknowledge that I am still part of this family. Remember me at special times.*

I went to hang Ron's robe in his closet one morning and the smell of his after shave, medicine he had taken, the worn leather smell from his old football and baseball glove, all mingled into an overpowering memory. My sense of smell screamed at my logical mind: *He's here!*

My arms went around the clothes as though holding Ron and I cried a deep sobbing, releasing flood of tears. When I finally stopped, I heard a sound behind me.

Sol had pulled the spread from the pillow and was clawing and purring wildly. It was pitiful to watch. He buried his face in the pillow, his claws working in frantic rhythm. It still had Ron's smell, and in his grief, Sol was doing exactly the same thing I'd done in the closet.

I sat on Ron's bed and held the sad little cat as Ron had held him so many times. The purring slowed to normal. He closed his eyes and snuggled against me. Occasionally a little paw would gently touch my face.

If any teen-age boys came to visit, Sol would stare into their face as though they might tell him where Ron was.

We tried to give Sol some extra love, but he continued to haunt Ron's room. He resumed his lonely vigil on Ron's bed—waiting.

I hadn't thought Sheba missed Ron until I was cleaning under the basement steps and felt something brush my hair. I raised up to see her swatting at me through the steps. This had been a boxing game between Sheba and Ron. He kept an old pair of leather gloves under the bottom step for this game because she played rough. I put on the gloves and boxed at her. She darted over and through steps slapping at me.

"He's gone Sheba. Games won't bring him back," I cried, beating the steps with my fists until I wore myself out. "Ask and you shall receive has limits, doesn't it, God? Everywhere I turn, someone tells me about a miracle cure You sent. Are Your cures reserved for special people? Ron was special."

I prayed for understanding and forgiveness for the awful guilt I carried. Guilt because I was angry at God and the doctors who, it seemed to me, had neglected to look for what seemed so plain to us.

Since the first doctor apparently wasn't smart enough to think of a biopsy, why hadn't God reminded him? It would have been easy for God to put the thought in the doctor's mind. But He hadn't. "Jesus," I prayed, "help me!" And like everyone else in this time of instant food, heat, cold and cash, I expected instant answers to my prayers. But God worked in His own time to show me His way.

Kathy's birthday was the next month. "I don't feel we should bother with a cake this year," she said. "It wouldn't seem right without Ronnie to . . ." She wiped the tears away, unable to finish.

"Ron wouldn't want that. You know how important birthdays were to him." I made a simple cake and invited a few of her friends on the block.

While they were eating, Roger started laughing. "Hey, Kath, do you remember the time Ron and I spilled punch on your new dress? You were mad and yelling, so Ron . . ." He stopped, embarrassed that he had mentioned it. "I'm sorry," he said, "I forgot."

"That's OK, Roger," I said. "We want to talk about him." Soon the conversation turned back to their childhood fun and fights.

There was something different about the group that day. It wasn't just the fact that Ron, their fun maker, wasn't there. Since the last party we'd had, before Ron became ill, most of them had become teen-agers. Now, death had taken one from their midst. Their carefree days of childhood were over.

I don't know how I spent some days. They're blank. But I did take down Ron's clothes. He had said to give them to a cousin who was working his way through college. That was when I found Ron's journal.

There were sketches of houses he would never build, the plans for a nursery that would never be, unfinished stories, poems and thoughts of an unfinished life. I wasn't alone anymore as I read:

> My parents worried about car wrecks, war and tomorrow. But my enemy wasn't on the highway

or some distant land. It was right here, waiting. God, 17 years hasn't been very long. I wanted more. But You didn't promise it would be easy—nor pain free. I know I'm in the shadow of death, and I will soon cross that chasm from this world to eternity.

About my family, God, as I walk through the valley, I hear them weep often. Please, don't let them cling to the past in search of me. Help them realize that because I am part of their past, I'll be a part of their future, too. Let them remember the good times, Lord. And remind them of your promise, that someday the circle will be unbroken.

I read on, fascinated by the way I seemed to pick up Ron's train of thought. A strange feeling, much like that of a mild sedative, came over me. Picking up a pencil, my hand started writing as though it had a mind of its own. It went on for several seconds, then stopped.

The message read:

> Please don't live in the past with me
> Or feel that you don't care.
> Every success that comes to you three
> I'll feel that I had a share.
>
> Since I have shared so much of your past
> I must share in your future, too.
> Remember I'm only a prayer away
> And as close as God to you.

I had heard of such things happening to great religious leaders, but not to common ordinary people. Although I had often felt the Holy Spirit near, especially during Ron's illness, I had never experienced anything like this. When I showed the writing to Martin and Kathy that night, it gave hope to our faltering trust and restored our faith.

Day after day, I sat at Ron's desk feeling the urgent need to write the messages that would break into my thoughts. Sometimes they came in dreams. At times it was an addition to something Ron had written or simply a rearrangement. A verse about the sunrise was alone, written on a scrap of paper he had used for a bookmark. One night I couldn't sleep and sat in his room thinking. The thought came to me to put that verse in the middle of a poem Ron had written about our state park. That's where it belonged. I often felt as though I was merely the tool being used to finish something important.

And then it stopped. Whatever had caused it was gone. I felt as empty as the night I discovered the tapes had been erased. One afternoon I sat in Ron's chair. I fell asleep and dreamed Ron was there. "I'm sorry I haven't been back lately," he said. "Remember the first summer I went to camp? It was so strange, I was lonely and called home. Then I adjusted to the place and everything was fine." As he moved away from me, I cried out and was startled by the sound of my voice.

Scripture tells about the influence of the Spirit of God upon the soul—extending to its sleeping as well as waking thoughts. The Book of Job mentions dreams and visions in sleep as the chosen method of God's revelation of himself to man.

The dream, or whatever it was, seemed to be the end. Depression replaced grief. Each time I would read about young people getting into trouble, I would cry out, "Lord, why did you take Ron?"

At one point I had felt depressed for days. I sat in Ron's room not answering the telephone or the door. Everyone's well meaning advice only made me angry. I could feel Ron was close to me with his rock collection, models of boats and airplanes—all the remarkable things a boy can collect in 17 years. And I resented intruders.

A soft knock at the door went unanswered. *No,* I thought, *company is the last thing I want!*

The knocking continued until I finally gave up. Jimmie, twisted and bent from a childhood disease, grasped the railing to steady his jerking body.

"Hello. I'll bet you didn't know I was able to be up again and selling for camp," he said, holding his basket out to me.

As I looked through the tiny assortment, I remembered he hadn't been by for a long time. We always bought from him although we usually didn't need what he was selling.

After Ron started high school, Jimmie would be waiting on his corner to talk. He was so thrilled about the ROTC and wanted to hear everything they did. Jimmie wasn't able to attend school and seemed to get enjoyment out of sharing Ron's experiences.

"Is Ron going to college next year?" Jimmie asked, looking past me. "Is he home?"

"Ron died in February."

He tried to steady his jerking body. "How? I mean, was it an accident?"

"No, he died of cancer," I said gently.

Jimmie looked down at his twisted legs. "It just doesn't seem right—a healthy guy like him. Why would God take him and . . ."

He blinked back tears. "Ron was always nice to me—making me part of his world. I did wonder why he didn't come by while I was ill. Mom said he was probably too busy. But he was my friend; I was sure he'd be there if he could."

We stood silent for a moment, then Jimmie broke into my thoughts. "Going to camp doesn't seem very important now."

"Please," I said, "Ron wouldn't want you to feel that way." Jimmie and I talked about Ron, about it almost being spring, and he promised to stop and visit each time he came our way. I paid him for the things I'd picked out. He went down the drive in his jerking, stumbling walk, then turned to wave.

I remembered Jesus' words: "I will not leave you comfortless: I will come to you" (John 14:18). And He had. Jimmie had just shown me that Ron had made his life happier. How many people had my son touched that I would never know about?

Jimmie, bless him, wasn't afraid to talk about Ron. I wanted to talk about him, but most people were ill at ease when his name was mentioned. We wanted to hear someone else say, "I'll miss him, too."

My mother had wanted to talk about Dad after he died. It seemed my family were the only ones who would let her. Others would change the subject as though Dad had never existed. Is this all a life means?

Many people were the same way with me. If I mentioned Ron in a conversation, they would become awkward and uneasy. Maybe they were afraid it would upset me—or was it the thought and finality of death that made them change the subject?

Jesus knew I needed comfort. He didn't choose to send it by way of a doctor or pastor. Comforting words came from one less fortunate—a boy who would no longer wait on a street corner to hear about an exciting world he could never take part in. A friend who was not afraid to say, "I'll miss him."

Epilogue

Spring came that year. I hadn't expected it. Somehow, I didn't think the world would continue exactly the same. Wild geese flew north. Ron's lilies were peeking through the ground. It seemed all life was going on except one.

I was working in the yard one morning when the sound of a child's voice startled me. "I could help you," he called. There stood four-year-old Tommy peering through the fence. As usual, his face was dirty, his hair ruffled, and his eyes pleaded desperately for someone to pay attention to him.

Tommy's dad was dead, his mother wasn't home much, and he was left in the care of an aunt who made him stay outside most of the day. They were new to the area so he didn't know how little boys made my heart ache.

"Some other time," I said. He didn't whine and argue

like many kids. With the air of one who was used to rebuffs, he walked slowly down the drive kicking imaginary rocks—or was it an unloving world he was kicking?

Trying to put all the Tommys of the world from my mind, I turned back to pulling the first tiny weeds from around the patio. As I thought of other spring days when children played in the yard, a land turtle came lumbering out of the shrubs. He stopped as though trying to make up his mind.

"Charley!" I said, moving over to him. "We didn't know you were still around." I rubbed my finger lightly on his head. He blinked and stuck his wrinkled neck out for some scratching. It was Charley.

Years before, the land behind our property had been a farm. We watched the city creep closer, as noisy machines chewed up trees and turned the farm into rows of look-alike houses on naked streets. Gradually, the little creatures that had lived there moved out of the way of progress. It was then Charley took up residence in our yard. It had everything a little turtle could want—a garden, fish pond and freedom.

Charley lost his freedom a few times when a big dog would carry what it thought was an odd shaped bone home to chew. We would bring him back none the worse for his experience. There were trips to school for "show and tell."

Slowpoke Charley could often be found in the middle of stomach games. Those are the games children play when they all sprawl out on their stomachs. He ruined many marble games, and was the star attraction when they played with the two-inch plastic soldiers, cowboys and Indians, and space men.

One day the boys had set up an elaborate "army." The attack of the good guys was led by General Charley.

His paddle-like legs waded through the enemy camp upsetting tents, tanks, and weapons carriers smaller than the leader.

"Is Charley supposed to be in there?" I asked.

Several faces peered up at me with those looks that seem to say, "Boy, moms sure don't know much, sometimes."

Ron decided to enlighten me. "You remember the Trojan horse don't you? Well, Charley is our Trojan turtle. He's better than a tank. When we play space men, Charley is a Martian giant. He can be a bull-dozer, too. Just like the ones that cleared the farm he lived on." Somehow I didn't think Charley would like that comparison.

I'm sure the turtle missed those games as his friends grew into teens. Once while spading the garden, Ron found Charley. "Hey, Kath," I heard him call, "come greet an old friend." For a long time they sat cross-legged on the ground playing with a part of their childhood memories.

"Remember . . . " I would hear one of them say. As they returned to their work, Kathy remarked, "Charley reminds me of Puff the Magic Dragon when the little kids no longer came to play with him."

Those were such good years—full of love and laughter. Now the house seemed so empty during the day. I stayed outside as much as I could. The flag on Ron's bed was a constant reminder he was away forever. And little boys like Tommy only brought back the pain of our loss.

Charley squirmed in my hands, bringing my thoughts back to the present. "Are you still a Trojan turtle?" I asked. "Another meaning is something intended to undermine from within. Did God send you to undermine my self-pity and make me start living again?"

Charley stretched his neck further out of his shell so I

could reach some unscratched spots. Even little turtles needed love.

Tommy stood at the curb looking forlornly down the street. "Maybe you *can* help me, Tommy," I called "In fact, I'm sure you will," I added as the eager child made a dash for my gate.

Tommy had never seen a turtle before, and was afraid at first. "He might bite!" he exclaimed.

I assured him Charley wouldn't bite, and he sprawled out on his stomach and looked Charley in the eye. "Hi, turtle, do you like me?"

Charley blinked and moved toward the edge of the patio. "Golly," Tommy said, "he doesn't like me, either." The child lay still, watching the turtle crawl off toward the garden.

I could feel Tommy's loneliness and feeling of rejection although he wasn't saying a word. "He doesn't know you yet. Give him time and he'll like you. Tell you what. As soon as I finish weeding I'll play with you."

"I'll help!" he said, eagerly pulling everything in sight.

"Let me show you what to pull first," I told him.

For the next hour, two lonely humans talked about turtles, why we pulled weeds, and playing ball.

Tommy helped me a lot that summer. I had started building a shell around my heart that was even harder than the one Charley retreated into.

There were times I envied Charley. If he felt the least bit threatened, all he had to do was withdraw into his shell and shut out the world. I tried to do that, and many times a grubby little boy would show up at my door asking, "Can you come out and play?"

Tommy followed me through the yard asking questions. One day he noticed ivy creeping along the rock wall. "How come that vine stays up on the wall? Even the wind doesn't blow it off."

I showed him the many little shoots or tendrils which had attached themselves to the rough rocks.

"If there was only one or just a few shoots they couldn't support the vine," I explained. "But there are many of them and each holds a little. By pulling together, they are able to support the heavy vine."

Tommy carefully examined the tendrils and exclaimed, "Just like us!"

"Like us?" I asked. "How do you mean?"

"Why, like me and you. You don't have a little boy to help you any more. And I don't have a grandma to tell me stories. So we help each other."

I gathered him in my arms and buried my face in his sweaty hair to hide my tears. It didn't work. A strong little hand patted my shoulder. "It's OK to cry. I do sometimes."

A few months later, Tommy's grandparents got custody of him. I rejoiced with him when he left for his new life in another state. It was lonely without him, but he had helped me through the bad months.

In the fall after Tommy left, I found Charley's empty shell under a bush. I buried it beside other pets. As I pressed the tiny flower bulbs into the wet earth over the new grave, it seemed as though I could hear all the children's laughter Charley brought to our yard. *Thank you, Lord, for a most fitting eulogy for a Trojan turtle. And thank you for sending him and Tommy when I needed them.*